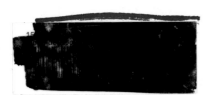

Motor
Development
Issues and Applications

Motor Development

ISSUES AND APPLICATIONS

Marcella V. Ridenour, *Temple University*
Jacqueline Herkowitz, *The Ohio State University*
Jane E. Clark, *University of Iowa*
Janet Teeple, *University of Illinois*
Mary Ann Roberton, *University of Wisconsin*

Edited by Marcella V. Ridenour

PRINCETON BOOK COMPANY, Publishers
Princeton, New Jersey

TABLE OF CONTENTS

INTRODUCTION

This book presents current issues and applications in the scholarly study of motor development of young children. The authors have brought together several unique approaches to this study. Prior books on motor development have emphasized the study of age-related physical growth and motor development trends. Although creating detailed descriptions of motor behavior is a necessary step in understanding motor development, however, it should not be considered the only significant field of study within motor development.

Part I of this book presents a theoretical model of growth and development which provides a frame-work for the critical growth factors associated with motor development.

In Part II we turn to specific *issues*. Contemporary issues in motor development, which are not included in Chapters 3 through 6, are briefly identified and summarized in Chapter 2. The issues included in this chapter are fetal development, childbirth, neonate and infant environments, neural control of movement, delays and disabilities, maternal and infant nutrition, early skill development programs, competitive sports, and perceptual-motor interrelationships. Chapter 3 first describes popular infant motor development programs, and then critiques these programs based on available research. Chapter 4 presents a summary of recent research documenting predictable stages in motor development. The literature in experimental, social, and developmental psychology during the past five years reflects an increased awareness of the importance of both sex role expectations and memory processes in the understanding of the developing child. Chapter 5 first examines the normative data describing sex differences on selected motor skills and then continues to describe the psychosociological interactions in early childhood that may influence these sex differences. Chapter 6 describes memory processes and applies these processes to the acquisition and retention of motor skills by young children. Sex role expectations and memory processes are underlying factors that relate to both parent and teacher behavior and the optimal development of motor skills.

In Part III the focus shifts to *applications* as divided into three broad concerns: *environments, curricula,* and *evaluation.* These three areas reflect the needs of the motor development specialist: environmental designs to enhance motor development, organization of curricula based on appropriate task analysis, and guidelines for the selection of evaluation instruments. Specifically, Chapter 7 presents a rationale for the design of playspaces, examines a variety of environmental elements, and describes techniques for evaluating the playspace. Chapter 8 provides an instructional approach to developmental task analysis, involving the design of sequentially ordered motor experiences and the identification of variables which limit or enhance the performance of a motor skill. Chapter 9 then presents six instruments for evaluating the status of motor development in children.

The editor, realizing that the reader of this book may have special interests not explored fully here, presents two appendices to provide guidance for future study, research, and practical experiences. Appendix A suggests step-by-step procedures for locating and retrieving literature on specialized topics within motor development. This appendix can assist undergraduate and graduate students searching the literature in motor development to present an original scholarly paper based on completed research.

Since the scope of the motor development laboratory is so interdisciplinary, usually an inexperienced coordinator will need suggestions on the purchase of tools and resources as well as potential activities for his or her motor development laboratory. Appendix B presents many suggestions regarding the organization, facilities, resources, and activities of a motor development laboratory. In addition, six examples of laboratory projects are described. These six laboratory projects can serve as models for undergraduate students, to assist them with the design and construction of their own projects. All play equipment described by Dr. Jacqueline Herkowitz in her discussion of the design of play-spaces for children could be built in the described motor development laboratory.

Only through the interaction of the library and laboratory can the valuable information in this book be applied to enhance the motor development of infants and young children.

Acknowledgments

We wish to acknowledge the invaluable assistance of the following people for their contributions to this book: Jeffrey Cook for the photography in Chapter 1; Edward Oppenheim for the photography in Chapter 3; Kahalil and Kobie Roberts, Danny and Meegan Fitzgerald, Michael Bressler, Alexis Asnin, and Sherri Rebecca Martin who served as models for the photographs in Chapter 3; the Ohio State Audiovisual Service for the photographs in Chapter 7, Gerald Gabow and Jenny Barone for the illustrations in Appendix B; Louis Garrozzo for designing and building the climbing boxes and sliding board in Appendix B; Tom Tomekovich for designing and building the wooden spool house in Appendix B; and Nora Boseman for her assistance with proofreading.

Part I

**Physical Growth
and Motor Development**

1

Physical Growth and Maturation

JANET TEEPLE

For many years physicians, physical educators, psychologists, and elementary educators have been interested in the motor development of children. Journals and books abound with articles discussing specific aspects of physical growth, physiological maturation, motor performance, and motor development. Unfortunately, this vast body of knowledge remains scattered and unfocused. To avoid further replication of the prevalent random "hit or miss" approach, we must develop a theoretical model of growth and motor development.

Motor Development Model

In this chapter we provide a framework which places the critical growth factors associated with motor development of children in a useful theoretical construct. But to do this we must first identify which kinds of factors are "change" phenomena and which kinds of factors are "status" phenomena. For purposes of introduction of the model, motor development, physical growth, and physiological maturation may be viewed as *change phenomena*. That is, these terms represent processes or developmental effects on the status factors. Motor performance, body size, and body composition could be considered *status factors*. These parameters represent a level of development, or the result of change, attained at any given time. For example, increases in body size resulting from the continuous processes of growth and maturation can be measured as the *status* of the child because at a given time on a given day a child will have a unique height and weight.

Status factors (such as motor performance, body size, and body composition) may be assessed once or over a series of time periods. The relationships of these components with each other can be statistically determined for any given time and the pattern of these status relationships across a series of test sessions can be plotted. In addition, the change phenomena can be measured by assessing differences in the same variables over several time periods. The influences of changes in one factor on changes in another factor can then be investigated. This second approach helps us to judge the real effect of our motor programs, health programs, or education programs on developing children. Such long-term investigations are quite expensive, however, so studies of this nature are rare. Most of our information then, comes from cross-sectionally designed studies, and we infer from them possible change effects. The model for motor development and growth presented here includes an attempt to accommodate both status and change kinds of designs and derivable information.

For this model, then, there are two main status factors: the *performer* and the *task* to be performed. The two change factors are *growth/maturation* and the *performer-task interaction*. These four basic components are shown in Figure 1-1. The meaning of the words rather than the shapes of the boxes are used to differentiate status and change factors.

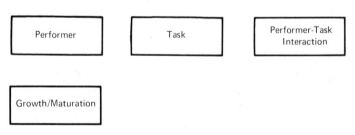

Figure 1-1.   Basic components of the motor development model.

For the sake of simplicity, *motor development* has been defined as "progressive change in motor performance." Thus, a model of its structure must include indications of the means of change. Figure 1-2 adds to the basic components the connectors or process labels to show logical relationships, among the parts. These processes are called *redefinition* of the task, *learning, stimulation/inhibition,* and *development.*

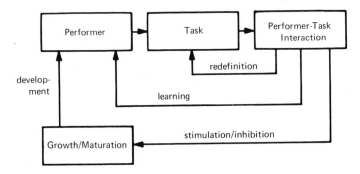

Figure 1-2. Relationships among the basic components of the motor development model.

Redefinition refers to the child's reaction to the task he has just performed. He may decide to change the task before his next performance to make it easier, more difficult, more complex, or different in some other way. In other words, he may change the goal or nature of the task itself.

Learning refers to changes in the child while he or she maintains the same goal of the task. The child may change some aspect of his technique of performance or, in the case of complex tasks, conquer some phase of the task. Developmentally, by interacting with the task, the child may perceive it differently or understand better the goals inherent in it. In terms of strength requirements of some tasks, increases in apparent strength may result from neurological learning rather than a muscle tissue change.

Stimulation/inhibition is a process affecting the rate of physical growth and, possibly, physiological maturation. This effect is not likely to be significant nor detectable after any single motor act, but is rather an effect built up over time. The inhibition component can be exemplified by laboratory animals subjected to intense forced exercise and limited diet which causes them to grow into smaller animals than their control litter mates. Similarly, in some cultures heavy manual labor involving carrying heavy weights results in compression on the ends of long bones and, eventually, shorter stature. Some minimal level of physical activity appears to be necessary to stimulate normal physical growth in children. This is evident in the atrophy which occurs when a limb is encased in a cast for a long time or when a child is confined to extended bed rest. Inhibition could also refer to loss of fat as a result of training programs and diets designed for weight loss in adults.

Some levels of activity appear to optimize physical growth (Malina, 1969); active children are frequently larger than their inactive peers. Hypertrophy of muscles does not occur in prepubescent children of either sex regardless of the type of training (Gifford, 1973).

Exercise, coupled with the genetically influenced normal growing pattern, results in a summative process labeled *development.* The product of the development process is the particular make up of the performer at any given time. Thus, the general characteristics of the child about to perform a task both influence his ability to perform this specific motor task and are influenced by his having performed other motor tasks.

As one more dimension of this hierarchical-process model, we should identify some of the factors which help to define and influence each of the basic components (see Figure 1-3). In fact, most of the growth and development research focuses on one or more of these defining factors rather than on the wholistic questions. Why? Because the total dynamics of the child in a movement setting are too complex when considered simultaneously in a single study.

As noted in Figure 1-3, what the performer brings to a task includes such parameters as body size, body composition (the fat and fat-free components), cardiorespiratory capacity, neurophysiological status, physical maturation level, social-cultural skills, and mental-cognitive capabilities. These factors describe the limits of his motor performance.

The task itself can be defined in terms of the kinetics, kinematics, neuromotor control, cardiorespiratory demands, and cognitive understanding necessary for its accomplishment. *Kinematics* and *kinetics* are technical terms referring to the mechanical components of speed, distance, angular displacement, and forces needed to perform a task. Similarly, some tasks require certain levels of quickness, steadiness, or exactness of submaximal force production which are a function of neuromotor control. Large cardiorespiratory demands are evidenced in endurance tasks, and cognitive understanding is required in varying amounts for all goal-directed movement. The child's performer descriptors must at least meet the task requirements if he or she is to be successful at the task.

Some results of the child interacting with the task are physical stress, emotional gratification, and psychomotor information. Motivation may be considered a combination of these results. The performer descriptors do not necessarily ensure successful performance, even if the performer has the individual capacities demanded in the task descriptors. The interaction of performer and task may be necessary for the child to improve his performance up to his physical limits by combinations of learning, redefinition, and stimulation/inhibition.

Regardless of the task, phylogenetic factors—such as genetic coding and mutation—and ontogenetic factors—such as nutrition, disease and injury, and emotional-social influences—can all influence the pattern and rate of growth and maturation. This process of development, in turn, affects the performer's potential for future motor performance. The whole model, with all its parts taken together, describes motor development.

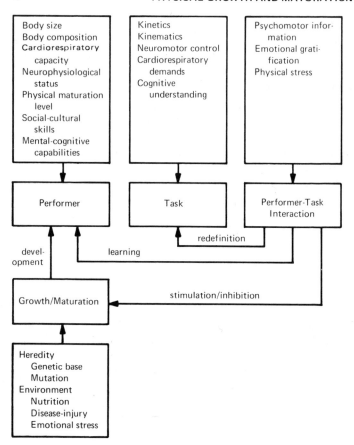

Figure 1-3. Factors influencing the basic components of the motor development model.

Normal Morphologic Growth

With this bioscience-oriented model in mind, let us now explore some of the information available about growth and the performer in terms of his motor performance capacity. Although some of our information is gleaned from animal studies and some from studies of children, we still have only a meager understanding of the complexities of motor development or normal physical growth and maturation. For example, studies dealing with adult body composition and motor performance cannot always be legitimately extrapolated directly to children. Indeed, it is crucial to understand the nature of growth in children.

The normal pattern of human growth is a nonlinear, fairly predictable, age-related phenomenon. The nonlinearity of growth patterns results in a physical structure for children which at any given age is simply not proportionally equivalent to a "scaleddown" adult. For example, nearly half of an adult's height can be attributed to leg length, while a child's leg is much less than one-half his total body height. The pattern of the rate of growth of the limbs exceeding the rate of growth of the trunk eventually results in the adult proportion (see Figure 1-4.) Similar discrepancies between adult and child body proportions are apparent in head size, arm lengths, shoulder and hip widths, and general morphological features (Meredith, 1939; Medawar, 1944; McCammon, 1970).

Since task success, and thus motor development, is at least in part a function of the mechanics of the task requirements, the implications of these disproportionate body size differences are evident. For example, the levers used for throwing, running, and kicking are disproportionately shorter in children than in adults (see Figures 1-5 to 1-7). Thus, it would be inappropriate to determine optimal movement patterns for children from biomechanics data taken from adults. Wickstrom's (1970) review clearly illustrates some of these differences for gross motor skills.

In addition, within very young age groups, body shape seems to account for some of the variability in the age of onset of various developmental motor skills. For example, Shirley (1931) and Bayley (1935) have shown that children with relatively long legs who are not overweight tend to walk earlier than children with proportionately shorter legs. This may be a maturation phenomenon coupled with other physiological development, but is interesting enough to warrant further study. In fact, we have very little hard data which indicate just how much of the timing of the onset of the so-called developmental milestones can be accounted for by simple morphological factors such as body proportions.

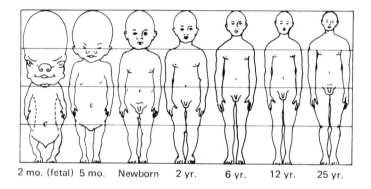

2 mo. (fetal) 5 mo.   Newborn   2 yr.   6 yr.   12 yr.   25 yr.

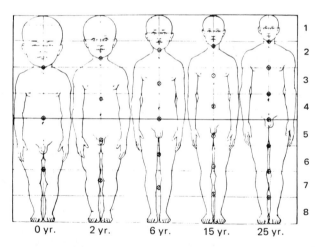

0 yr.   2 yr.   6 yr.   15 yr.   25 yr.

Figure 1-4. Prenatal and postnatal body proportion changes. The upper diagram illustrates general prenatal and postnatal structural growth. Changes in body proportion as a function of head size are illustrated in the lower diagrams. (From Scammon, R. E., 1927, with permisssion from Timiras, P. S. *Developmental Physiology and Aging.* New York: Macmillan, 1973.

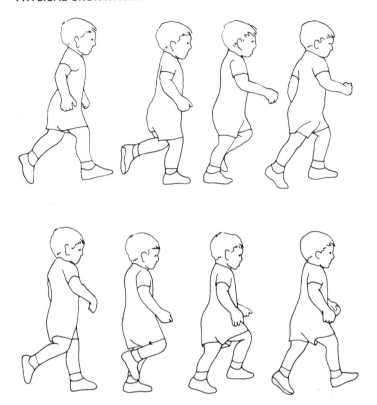

Figure 1-5. Running style of an 18-month-old child.

Not only the immediate body size but also the *pattern of change or growth* may affect motor development. Height and weight, for example, undergo fluctuatig periods of very rapid and very slow increase. The slow and spurt phases of normal growth can be seen by plotting the differences in height or weight from year to year, rather than the accumulated height and weight. This curve is called a *velocity curve,* and indicates the rate of change of size. The *acceleration curve* shows the rate of change in velocity. Small changes in the rate of growth are amplified and show more clearly the growth patterns at various ages

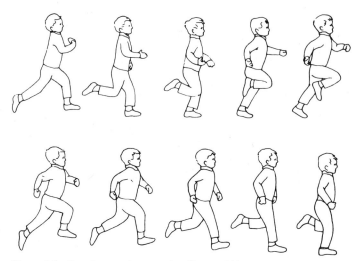

Figure 1-6. Running at a fast pace in a 3-year-old boy.

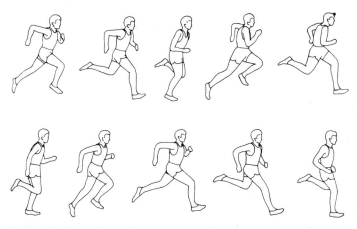

Figure 1-7. Mature form in running at a sprint pace. Note the change in stride length and use of arms from 18 months to adult pattern. (Figs. 1.5-1.7 from Wickstrom, R. *Fundamental Motor Patterns,* Philadelphia: Lea & Febiger, 1970, with permission.)

(see Figure 1-8). The adolescent height increase is evident as a growth spurt (Shuttleworth, 1939 as cited in Tanner, 1962). There is little definitive research which suggests the extent to

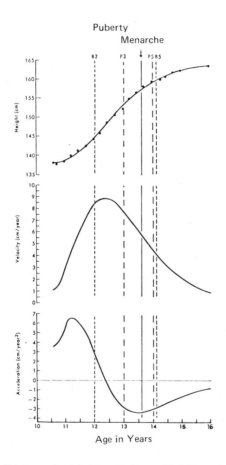

Figure 1-8. Height attained, height velocity, and height acceleration curves of a girl at adolescence. *B2* marks beginning breast development, *B5* adult form. *P3* marks intermediate stage of pubic hair development, *P5* adult form. (From Maclaren, A., ed. *Advances in Reproductive Physiology,* Vol. 2. London: Elek Books, 1967, with permission.)

which these patterns affect motor performance (Espenschade and Eckert, 1967; Eichorn, 1970; Rarick, 1973). Figure 1-9 shows the earlier acceleration in height for girls and the greater peak acceleration for boys. Another interesting pattern of growth is that associated with seasonal cycles (see Figure 1-10). Weight gains in children appear to be greater in autumn, while height gains are greater in spring (Tanner, 1961). These growth patterns probably result from dietary and activity patterns of people living in areas with distinct seasonal climates. Again, the implications of this pattern of growth have not been adequately explored yet.

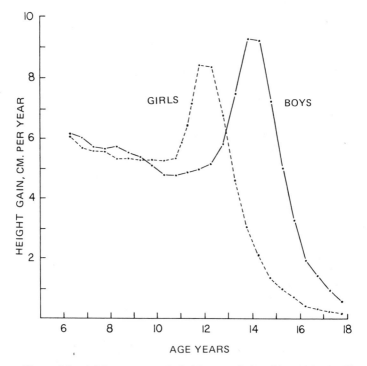

Figure 1-9. Adolescent spurt in height growth for girls and boys. The curves are from subjects who have their peak velocities during the model years 12 to 13 for girls, and 14 to 15 for boys. (Data from Shuttelworth, 1939. Reprinted with permission from Tanner, J. *Growth at Adolescence,* 2nd ed. Oxford: Blackwell Scientific Publications, Ltd., 1962.)

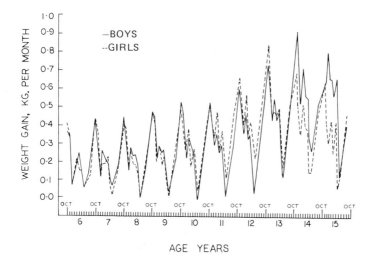

Figure 1-10. Seasonal variation of weight gains in boys and girls of V.S. P.H.S., Hagerstown Survey, 1921-1928. (Redrawn from Palmer, 1933. Reprinted with permission from Tannner, J. *Growth at Adolescence,* 2nd ed. Oxford: Blackwell Scientific Publications, Ltd., 1962.)

There are also typical growth patterns for internal organs and systems. Figure 1-11 shows the classical work of Scammon (1930), who weighed organs of fetuses and children who had died of non-dissipating causes. These patterns further substantiate the concept that a child is not simply a miniature adult. Scammon's work indicates that the extremely rapid prenatal growth patterns are nearly parallel. After birth, however, several distinct patterns of weight gain emerge. Note, for example, the familiar general body curve associated with bone, muscle, and total body weight. These parameters derive from the same embryonic germ layer, the mesoderm. In contrast, the nervous system, lymphatic system, and reproductive system all have uniquely different patterns of development. Looking at this graph for, let's say, a 5-year-old child, note that each system has progressed to a different point in terms of a 20-year-old terminal standard. Thus, although the 5-year-old is 25 percent the chronological age of the 20-year-old, each of his systems has not attained 25 percent of the adult weight. Should we, then, expect him to perform at 25 percent of his adult motor performance level?

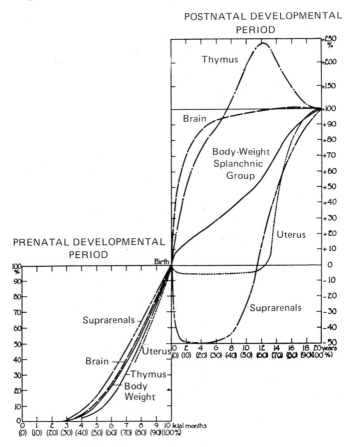

Figure 1-11. Diagram showing growth in weight of the human body and organs during prenatal and postnatal life. The abscissa indicates age and the ordinate the size attained in percentage of final weight (taken as 100 percent) reached at birth or at 20 years. (Modified from Scammon, 1930, with permission from Timiras, P. S. *Developmental Physiology and Aging.* New York: Macmillan, 1973.

Physiological Maturation

Coupled with the concept of growth, or increase in size, is the concept of maturation. This very elusive term refers to how far a child has progressed in quality of physiological status in light of his genetically predetermined adult status. Both growth and maturation are genetically and environmentally influenced; both refer to cellular, organ, and system development; and both are uniquely different yet inseparable from each other (Falkner, 1966; Klissouras, 1973).

Maturation is frequently differentiated from growth by reference to quality of biochemical makeup rather than size alone. For example, *x*-rays of growing bones indicate the amount of calcification that has occurred, allowing one to disregard, essentially, the actual size of the bones. Figure 1-12 shows an adult hand and wrist, with calcification completed and the epiphyses fused with the shaft of the bones. Figures 1-13 to 1-15 show hand *x*-rays of progressively younger children. The spaces where the wrist bones should be are simply cartilaginous bones not yet calcified and, thus, not yet radio-opaque. The growth lines between the epiphyses and the shaft of the long bones are also cartilaginous and not calcified.

Various systems of estimating skeletal age or maturation of the skeletal system have been devised (Tanner *et al.*, 1962; Pyle, 1971; Clark & Hayman, 1962) and debated (*American Journal of Physical Anthropology,* November, 1971). The basic idea is that skeletal maturation provides more information about the developmental status of the child than does chronological age. Chronological age has a constant increment: 1 calendar year for 1 year of age. Maturation, on the other hand, does not follow such a straight-line developmental curve. A child may increase in maturation 2 years during the same year that he increases in chronological age only 1 year. Similarly, 1 chronological year may result in only ½ year gain in normative skeletal maturation. As Figure 1-16 illustrates, there are differences in the ages of peak velocity of growth. These individual differences in maturation are normal just as individual differences in mature overall body size are normal.

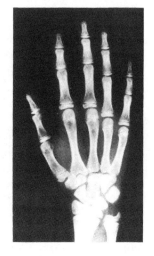

Figure 1-12. *X*-ray of hand. Skeletal ages: Male—156 months, female—128 months. (From Pyle, S.I.) *A Radiographic Standard of Reference for the Growing Hand and Wrist.* Copyright © 1971 by Year Book Medical Publishers, Inc., Chicago, with permission.

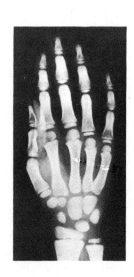

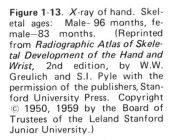

Figure 1-13. *X*-ray of hand. Skeletal ages: Male- 96 months, female—83 months. (Reprinted from *Radiographic Atlas of Skeletal Development of the Hand and Wrist,* 2nd edition, by W.W. Greulich and S.I. Pyle with the permission of the publishers, Stanford University Press. Copyright © 1950, 1959 by the Board of Trustees of the Leland Stanford Junior University.)

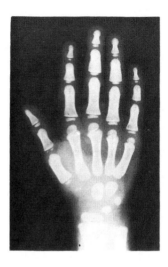

Figure 1-14. *X*-ray of hand. Skeletal ages: Male—48 months, female—37 months. (From Pyle, S.I.) *A Radiographic Standard of Reference for the Growing Hand and Wrist.* Copyright © 1971 by Year Book Medical Publishers, Inc., Chicago, with permission.

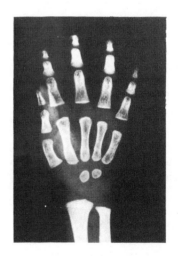

Figure 1-15. *X*-ray of hand. Skeletal ages: Male—12 months, female—10 months. (From Pyle, S.I.) *A Radiographic Standard of Reference for the Growing Hand and Wrist.* Copyright © 1971 by Year Book Medical Publishers, Inc., Chicago, with permission.

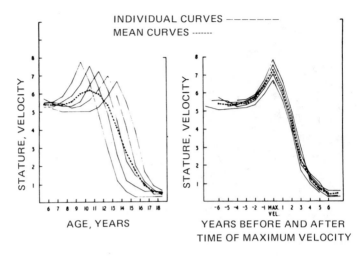

Figure 1-16. Relation between individual and mean velocities during the adolescent spurt. In the left diagram height gains are plotted against chronological age; in the right curve they are plotted according to their time of maximum velocity. (Data from Shuttleworth, 1937. Reprinted with permission from Tanner, J. *Growth at Adolescence,* 2nd ed. Oxford: Blackwell Scientific Publications, Ltd., 1962.)

Skeletal maturation is thought to reflect maturation of other physiological systems and has the advantage of discernible change throughout all the growing years. Other ways of assessing maturation, suitable for restricted age ranges, include dental eruption (Tanner, 1962; Demirjian *et al.*, 1973) and secondary sex-characteristics assessment (Tanner, 1962; Young, 1963, 1968). It is interesting to note that although maturation rates do differ among children, their overriding pattern of development is very similar, differing primarily in the chronological ages at which certain maturation phases occur.

Many other anthropometric parameters grow in relation to maturation rather than age (Agarwal *et al.*, 1974). The reasons for the chronological age differences is not totally clear yet; but factors such as genetics, hormones, nutrition, disease, and emotional stress appear to play important roles (Acheson, 1966).

Implications for Children's Programs

One major implication of motor development which can be drawn from the understanding of age differences in the attainment of physical growth levels is a redirecting of standards for motor development levels. For example, many pediatricians, parents, and people who work with preschool children will still use Shirley's 1933 chronological standards (see Figure 1-17) for determining whether or not a child is "developing normally," even though data from the same author (Shirley, 1931) indicated that body composition and size play a major role in determining the age of onset of these motor milestones (see discussion in Espenschade and Eckert, 1967). On the other hand, it would be inappropriate to require hand-wrist x-rays of all preschoolers and elementary school students each year just to assess maturation status. At this point, it seems best to suggest that adults working with children be cognizant of normal growth and maturation patterns and deviations and derive expected behavioral levels based on this understanding. Additionally, children whose growth patterns deviate from normal, expected variability could be referred to appropriate health professionals. This action might result in early treatment and prevent long-range difficulties.

Most of what has been discussed about growth, maturation, and motor development is based on descriptive data, particularly data descriptive of white, middle-class children. We can describe growth and related changes, but we do not yet have a clear understanding of how and why development proceeds as it does. Investigations into the explanations of physical development are generally oriented to biochemical responses of various organs to hormones and cell metabolites produced or inhibited by genetic and environmental factors (Cheek, 1968; Cheek *et al.*, 1970; Timiras, 1973). For example, increase in muscle mass and fat mass are controlled by heredity, insulin, growth hormone, and sex hor-

mones interacting with nutrition (Cheek, 1971) and activity
(Parizkova, 1973; Edgerton, 1973). Malnutrition and undernutri-
tion affect all phases of growth and development because of influence on the nervous system (Cravioto, 1963, 1966). Motor development has been only incidentally studied in these investigations
with young children.

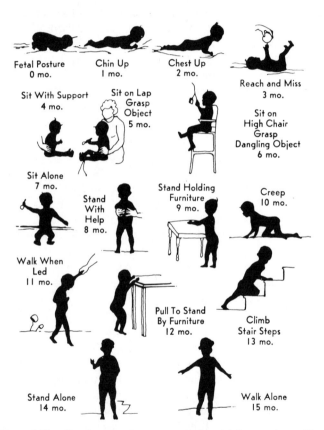

Figure 1-17. Developmental sequence in bipedal locomotion. (From
Shirley, M. M. *The First Two Years. A Study of Twenty-Five Babies,
vol. 2, Intellectual Development.* Minneapolis: University of Minnesota
Press, 1933, with permission of the publishers.)

Childhood diseases and extreme inactivity such as prescribed bed rest retard physical development. When these negative influences are removed, a phenomenon called *catch-up growth* occurs. This phenomenon is a metabolic rate increase which brings the child back up to where he would have been had he not been sick (Tanner, 1962). Catch-up growth is not totally effective if the retarding influences act for too long a time. No one has studied motor performance changes during these unique growth periods.

Finally, many of us still believe the fallacy that the cardiovascular system in children is not adequately developed for strenuous exercise; thus, children should be protected from possible heart damage by restricting their level of physical activity. This belief is founded on a scientific error made in 1879 (Beneke as cited in Karpovich, 1937) and popularized in a 1923 health textbook. The thought was that the arteries near the heart did not increase in size at the same rate as the heart itself. Karpovich refuted this claim in 1937, but a popular child development textbook published as recently as 1967 (Hurlock) still contains this misconception. Since the heart and circulation are derived from the same embryonic germ layer as muscle, and since skeletal muscle is the primary oxygen demand site during physical activity, it is logical to suspect that the cardiovascular system develops in the same growth pattern as the general body growth pattern described by Scammon (1930) and shown in Figure 1-4. Unfortunately youngsters have been over-protected for many generations because of a simple calculation error. On the other hand, children should not be forced into sudden or extreme activity without adequate preparation any more than adults should. Given common sense precautions, however, children clearly exhibit adequate cardiorespiratory responses to physical stress (Boas, 1931; Robinson, 1938, Astrand, 1952; Gifford, 1973; Bailey, 1976.)

Studies dealing with the positive effects of training on children's growth, body composition, and cardiorespiratory capacity are difficult to interpret. We like to think that physical activity programs increase physical fitness and increase motor performance capabilities. Data from very recent evaluations of the 12-minute run performances of young Brazilian children made first before the school system offered any physical education program, and then after a year of the newly instituted program (Matsudo, 1975), provide strong evidence in favor of positive gains resulting from such a program. As in most longitudinal studies, however, these children also grew in body size, which confounds the picture. Studies should indicate performance differences corrected for growth changes if they are to ascertain true programmatic effects. This was done by Parizkova (1973), who showed an increase in maximal and oxygen intake capacity as a function of age or growth for both active and inactive experimental groups over a 5-year period. When total body weight and muscle growth were considered, the cardiorespiratory differences between groups was still evident, although the changes over the years were not as striking for any of the groups. Clearly, researchers need to be careful to separate training effects from simple growth effects by obtaining ample growth data (Malina, 1969), especially when dealing with prepubescent children.

In short, although hundreds of studies have been completed dealing with growth and motor development of children, only a few people (Espenschade and Eckert, 1967; Rarick, 1973; and Corbin, 1973) have attempted to organize and integrate what we do know so that we can identify where we need to go next. It is hoped that the working model presented here will help to order the important but diverse literature in the motor development domain. Obviously we cannot study simultaneously all the critical factors associated with motor development in a single project, yet we must have some perspective of the factors that are studied before we can understand the real significance of each question.

REFERENCES

Acheson, R. Maturation of the skeleton. In Falkner, F., ed. *Human Development.* Philadelphia: Saunders, 1966.

Agarwal, K., *et al.* Physical growth characteristics in relation to sexual growth. *Indian Pediatrics,* 1974, *11,* 99-105.

American Journal of Physical Anthropology, November, 1971.

Astrand, P. *Experimental Studies of Working Capacity in Relation to Sex and Age.* Copenhagen: Munksgoaard, 1952.

Bailey D. A. The growing child and the need for physical activity. In Albinson, J., & Andrew, G., eds. *Child in Sport and Physical Activity.* Baltimore: University Park Press, 1976.

Bayley, N. The development of motor abilities during the first three years. *Monographs of the Society for Research in Child Development,* 1935, *1, 1-26.*

Boas, E. The heart rate of boys during and after exhaustive exercise. *Journal of Clinical Investigation,* 1931, *10,* 145.

Cheek, D. Hormonal and nutritional factors influencing muscle cell growth. *Journal of Dental Research,* 1971, *50,* 1385-1391.

Cheek, D. *Human Growth: Body Composition, Cell Growth, Energy and Intelligence.* Philadelphia: Lea & Febiger, 1968.

Cheek, D., *et al.* Cellular growth: nutrition and development. *Pediatrics,* 1970, *45,* 315-334.

Clark, H., & Hayman, H. Reduction of bone assessments necessary for the skeletal age determination of boys. *Research Quarterly,* 1962, *33,* 202-207.

Corbin, C. *A Textbook of Motor Development.* Dubuque: Brown, 1973.

Cravioto, J. Application of newer knowledge of nutrition on physical and mental growth and development. *American Journal of Public Health,* 1963, *55,* 1805.

Cravioto, J. Complexity of factors involved in protein-calorie malnutrition. *Bibliotheca Nutritio et Dieta,* 1970, *14,* 7-22.

Cravioto, J., *et al.* Nutrition, growth and neurointegrative development: an experimental and ecologic study. *Pediatrics,* 1966, *38,* 319.

Demirjian, A., *et al.* A new system of dental age assessment. *Human Biology,* 1973, *45,* 211-227.

Edgerton, V. R. Exercise and the growth and development of muscle tissue. In Rarick, G., ed. *Physical Activity: Human Growth and Development.* New York: Academic Press, 1973.

Eichorn, D. Physiological development. In Mussen, P., ed. *Carmichael's Manual of Child Psychology.* New York: Wiley, 1970.

Espenschade, A., & Eckert, H. *Motor Development.* Columbus: Merrill, 1967.

Falkner, F. *Human Development.* Philadelphia: Saunders, 1966.

Gifford, P. The effects of high resistance and high repetition physical activity on the body composition of prepubescent boys (Doctoral dissertation, University of Illinois, 1973). *Dissertation Abstracts International,* 1974, *35,* 243-A (University Microfilms No. 74-12, 022).

Greulich, W. W., & Pyle, S. I. *Radiographic Atlas of Skeletal Development of the Hand and Wrist, 2nd ed.* Stanford: Stanford University Press, 1959.

Hurlock, E. *Adolescent Development.* New York: McGraw-Hill, 1967.

Karpovich, P. Textbook fallacies regarding the development of the child's heart. *Research Quarterly,* 1937, *8,* 33.

Klissouras, V. Genetic aspects of physical fitness. *Journal of Sports Medicine and Physical Fitness,* 1973, *13,* 164-170.

Maclaren, A. (ed.) *Advances in Reproductive Physiology,* vol. 2 London: Elek Books, 1967.

Malina, R. Exercise as an influence upon growth-review and critique of current concepts. *Clinical Pediatrics,* 1969, *8,* 16-26.

Matsudo, V. Personal communication, May, 1975.

McCammon, R. *Human Growth and Development.* Springfield: Thomas, 1970.

Medawar, P. The shape of the human being as a function of time. *Proceedings of the Royal Society of London* (B), 1944, *132,* 133-141.

Meredith, H. Length of head and neck, trunk, and lower extremities of Iowa City children aged 7-17 years. *Child Development,* 1939, *10,* 129-144.

Parizkova, J. Body composition and exercise. In Rarick, G., ed. *Physical Activity: Human Growth and Development.* New York: Academic Press, 1973.

Pyle, S. I. *A Radiographic Standard of Reference for the Growing Hand and Wrist.* Chicago: Year Book Medical Publishers, 1971.

Rarick, G., ed. *Physical Activity: Human Growth and Development.* New York: Academic Press, 1973.

Robinson, S. Experimental studies of physical fitness in relation to age. *Arbeitsphysiologie,* 1938, *10,* 251-323.

Scammon, R. E. The first seriatim study of human growth. *American Journal of Physical Anthropology*, 1927, *10*, 329-336.

Scammon, R. E. The measurement of the body in childhood. In Harris, J.A., Jackson, C.M., Paterson, D.G., & Scammon, R.E. *The Measurement of Man*. Minneapolis: University of Minnesota Press, 1930.

Shirley, M. M. *The First Two Years, A Study of Twenty-Five Babies, vol. 1, Postural and Locomotor Development*. Minneapolis: University of Minnesota Press, 1931.

Shirley, M. M. *The First Two Years, A Study of Twenty-Five Babies, vol. 2, Intellectual Development*. Minneapolis: University of Minnesota Press, 1933.

Shuttleworth, F. The physical and mental growth of girls and boys age six to nineteen in relation to age at maximum growth. *Monographs of the Society for Research in Child Development*, 1939, *4* (3).

Tanner, J. *Education and Physical Growth*. London: University of London Press, 1961.

Tanner, J. *Growth at Adolescence*, 2nd ed. Oxford: Blackwell Scientific Publications, Ltd., 1962.

Tanner, J., & Taylor, G. *Growth*. New York: Time-Life Books, 1971.

Tanner, J., et al. *A New System for Estimating Skeletal Maturity from the Hand and Wrist*. Paris: International Children's Centre, 1962.

Timiras, P. S. *Developmental Physiology and Aging*. New York: MacMillan, 1973.

Wickstrom, R. *Fundamental Motor Patterns*. Philadelphia: Lea & Febiger, 1970.

Young, H. Aging and adolescence. *Developmental Medicine and Child Neurology*, 1963, *5*, 451-460.

Young, H., et al. Evaluation of physical maturity at adolescence. *Developmental Medicine and Child Neurology*, 1968, *10*, 338-348.

Part II

**Issues
in Motor Development**

2

Contemporary Issues
in Motor Development

MARCELLA V. RIDENOUR

The four key issues selected for in-depth examination in Part II, have been frequently researched, summarized, critiqued, and debated in publications associated with the study of motor development. There are however, many other issues in motor development, and we shall touch on several of these in this chapter.

One very interesting, and increasingly accurate study is that of fetal behavior. New instrumentation using ultrasound permits prenatal observation of the fetus almost as if it were on a television screen. Longitudinal studies of both physical and motor development may start with the fetus, rather than the newborn infant, providing details on the influence of prenatal maternal drugs, alcohol, disease, or activity level of the present or future motor and physical development of the fetus.

Another relevant issue is the effect of obstetric medication or natural childbirth on the physical and motor development of the infant. This issue is immediately followed by discussions on the advantages and disadvantages of first placing the newborn infant in an environment that simulates the maternal womb, and then gradually introducing him or her to home conditions (Leboyer, 1975). The values of vestibular, auditory, tactual, and visual stimulation of the newborn infant have been debated by child development authorities. For instance, some authorities recommend controlled vestibular stimulation, while others feel that even limited shaking may cause damage to the central nervous system resulting in potential brain damage interfering with the infant's development (Clark et al., 1977; Cherry, 1975).

Other researchers are concerned with identifying the electrochemical neural structures and their functions in developing the neural control of movement (Herman *et al.*, 1976; Taub, 1976; Szekely, 1976). These researchers are specialists in physiological psychology and developmental neurophysiology. Their research, usually involves implanting electronic sensors, administering chemical inhibitors, and performing surgery to observe the structure and functions of neural control systems as they relate to the development of movement behavior. As a result, their experiments are generally limited to animals.

Many applied motor development specialists are interested in the cause, effect, and treatment of motor development delays (Whiting, 1975; Lewko, 1976). During the past few years, they have emphasized early intervention for high-risk categories of infants, such as those with extremely young mothers, premature births, low birth weights, or genetic defects. Cross-cultural studies are continually providing new findings indicating the influence of the mother and infant's nutrition, physical environment, and socio-economic conditions on the cognitive and physical growth of the infant (Erishin, 1976). Emphasis here is on preventing delays in the acquisition of motor skills — or at least identifying and working with them as quickly as possible.

The influence of the infant's environment on motor development has been debated throughout this century. Generally, as biomedical engineers have developed more precise and accurate instrumentation for measuring both the onset and quality of motor skills, experiments have indicated greater influences of the environment on the performance of motor skills. Until a little over 10 years ago, the onset of infant walking was usually recorded only by the age of the first successful walking steps. An exception to this generalization is the excellent research by McGraw around 1940 (McGraw, 1940, 1945). Now, through the use of high-speed motion film records transformed to a computer by a digitizer, detailed movement organization records can describe the temporal and spatial relationships of body segments within the infant's walking pattern (Grieve *et al.*, 1976; Adrian, 1973;

Miller & Nelson, 1973; Roberts, 1971; Moore, 1977). These new procedures quickly provide accurate information on the quality and form of the infant's pre-walking and walking pattern.

Prior studies investigating only the onset (age of initial walking) have frequently indicated no significant differences for selected environmental conditions (Dennis, 1935, 1940). The use of a three-dimensional computer-assisted analysis of movement quality may reverse the early findings, which were based on limited data describing only the onset of the motor skills. The generally accepted classical studies investigating the relationships between the infant's environment and his initial acquisition of motor skills should be replicated using precise instrumentation to study the infant's movement patterns. In addition to replication studies, future research should investigate potential environmental influences on motor development in American homes. What have we created through excessive use of passive motion (strollers and automobile seats), playpens, walkers, plastic infant seats, and television? The results of these experiments would interest not only researchers but also, education classes and even popular periodicals.

Another issue has arisen with the physiological and biomechanical assessment tools and techniques which assist the sport specialist in selecting and training athletes. One technique used to examine athletic potential is a muscle biopsy to determine the ratio of slow-twitch (fatigue-resistant) and fast-twitch (rapid contraction with a high peak tension (Kevl et al, 1972; Edgerton, 1973). A runner with predominantly slow twitch fibers may be encouraged to participate in the long distance events, while a runner with predominantly fast-twitch fibers may be placed in the shorter running events. The complete effect of the interaction of heredity and training on fiber ratios has not yet been determined. Other similar biomechanical and physiological tests are also being used to predict athletic potential. Can you imagine a future where large-scale evaluations would identify children with desirable combinations of motor skills and physical characteristics? These elite children might be placed in summer or year-round

sport centers staffed with coaches, psychiatrists, exercise physio-
logists, motor learning specialists, and biomedical engineers who
would jointly determine the scientific training programs to develop athletic potential for participation in future national and
international competitions.

The influence of intensive athletic training and competition
on a child's development has been discussed at recent physical
education conferences. A national conference dealing with the
child in sports was held in Milwaukee, Wisconsin, in 1976 (Magill,
1977). Extensive discussions were held on the positive and negative consequences of competitive sports for children.

We do not have enough information to determine whether a motor skills program emphasizing general basic movement skills is
superior to programs emphasizing one group of sports skills. Possibly there may be an age-shift — indicating the advantages of an initial general movement program, followed later by sports-specific
programs. A new national franchise specializes in selling instructional packets for teaching tennis to 3-, 4-, and 5-year-old children.
The instructional packet includes a teacher workshop, modified
equipment, and lesson plans. Similar sports-specific programs are
available in dance forms, swimming, or gymnastics for preschool
children. Usually motor skill transfer is limited to skills involving
the same or similar movements.

The superiority of sports-specific instructional programs for
adults is generally recognized, but young children may benefit
from a basic movement program, especially if, after sport-
specific programs, they have trouble changing sports at a later
age, or if they have no opportunity to develop a variety of life-
long recreational skills. Most preschool and elementary physical
education programs asume that motor generalizations and fundamental motor skill learning will easily transfer to later acquisition of more specialized motor skill. On the other hand, research
must be completed to indicate the relationships between general
and specific motor skill programs in relation to the age and goals
of the child. Appropriate information should be available to
children and parents describing the social, psychological, and
physical effects of intense athletic training in a selected sport be-

fore they invest heavily in equipment, coaching, or travel. Independent investigations of public and private sports organizations should inform parents and children of potential psychological, physical, or financial abuses.

To describe interactions influencing the acquisition of motor skills, the perceptual and motor characteristics of movement skills must be examined and manipulated jointly. For example, today two groups of experimenters are investigating ball skills. One group is studying perceptual characteristics of a simulated ball environment using a fine motor response such as a key press or verbal response (Herkowitz, 1972; Ridenour, 1975; Whiting & Hutt, 1974); while the second group carefully analyzes fundamental motor skills, but makes no attempt to investigate the visual, or auditory, input to the child from the moving ball and its respective background (Victors, 1961). Yet high-speed cameras and electromechanical sensors permit continuous recording during initial acquisition trials of a motor skill. Not only can a three-dimensional image of the child's moving body be easily stored and retrieved from computer storage; but simultaneously his or her visual search strategy (represented by the location of eye movements and eye fixations during a motor task) may be stored and retrieved from the same computer storage (Bard & Fleury, 1976).

In studying these skills, researchers can ask, does the amount of time a child visually fixates on a moving ball increase or decrease as he becomes more skilled at catching or striking? Does a child with a motor performance decrement simultaneously have a decrement in the visual processes necessary for an accurate motor response? The monitoring of children's visual search patterns during the acquisition of motor skills will provide feedback to the teacher regarding the influence of the visual environment on this acquisition. Problems involving visual and auditory environments for motor skills can be easily investigated, and the findings can be applied to the design of environments for early skill acquisition. This *joint* examination of perceptual characteristics and movement organization will provide information to design optimal teaching environments for developmental movement activities.

Numerous interdisciplinary issues in motor development confront us. While those selected for Part II are limited to some of the more urgent issues, other questions can be identified—and possibly resolved—using the library sources described in Appendix A, or through experimental research in a motor development laboratory such as that described in Appendix B.

REFERENCES

Adrian, M. J. Cinematographic, electromyographic, and electrogoniometric techniques for analyzing human movements. In Wilmore, J. H. ed., *Exercise and Sports Science Reviews, Volume I,* New York: Academic Press, 1973, 343-350.

Bard, C., & Fleury, M. Analysis of visual search activity during sport problem situations. *Journal of Human Movement Studies,* 1976, *3,* 214-222.

Cherry, R. Spare the exercise, spoil the infant. *New York Times Magazine* February 9, 1975, 65-66. 69, 96.

Clark, L., Krevtzberg, J. R., & Chee. F. K. Vestibular stimulation influence on motor development. *Science,* 1977, *196,* 1228-1229.

Dennis, W. The effect of restricted practice on the reaching, sitting, and standing of two infants. *Journal of Genetic Psychology,* 1935, *47,* 17-32.

Dennis, W., & Dennis, M. G. The effect of cradling practice on the age of walking in Hopi children. *Journal of Genetic Psychology,* 1940, *56,* 77-96.

Edgerton, R. V. Exercise and the growth and development of muscle tissue. In Rarick, G. L., ed., *Physical Activity: Human Growth and Development,* New York: Academic Press, 1973, 1-31.

Erishin, H. Interaction of diverse social and biological influence on early development. Audiotape recorded at the 142nd Annual Meeting of the American Association for Advancement of Science, Boston, 1976.

Grieve, D. W., *et al. Techniques for the Analysis of Human Movement.* Princeton, N. J., Princeton Book Company, Publishers, 1976.

Herkowitz, J. Moving embedded figures test. *Research Quarterly,* 1972, 43, 479-488.

Herman, R. M., *et al.* eds. *Neural Control of Locomotion.* New York: Plenum Press, 1976.

John, E. R., *et al.* Neurometrics. *Science,* 1977, *196,* 1393-1410.

Kevl, J., Doll, E., & Keppler, D. *Energy Metabolism of Human Muscle.* Baltimore: University Press, 1972.

Leboyer, F. *Birth Without Violence.* New York: Random House, 1975.

Lewko, J. H. Current practices in evaluating motor behavior of disabled children. *The American Journal of Occupational Therapy,* 1976, *30,* 413-419.

Magill, R. A. Youth sports: an interdisciplinary view of readiness and effects. *Journal of Health, Physical Education, and Recreation,* 1977, *48,* 56-57.

McGraw, M. B. Neuromuscular development of the human infant as exemplified in the achievement of erect locomotion. *Journal of Pediatrics,* 1940, *17,* 747-771.

McGraw, M. B. *Neuromuscular Maturation of the Human Infant.* New York: MacMillan, 1945.

Miller, D. I., & Nelson, R. C. *Biomechanics in Sport: A Research Approach.* Philadelphia: Lea and Febiger, 1973.

Monty, R. A. *Eye Movements and Psychological Processes,* Hillsdale, N. J.: Lawrence Erlbaum Associates, Publisher, 1976.

Moore, K. Gideon's Magic Machine. *Sports Illustrated,* August 22, 1977, *47* (8), 52-60.

Ridenour, M. V. Influence of object size, speed, and direction on the perception of a moving object. *Research Quarterly,* 1975, *45,* 293-301.

Roberts, E. Cinematography in biochemical investigation. In Cooper, J. M., *Selected Topics in Biomechanics,* Chicago: The Athletic Institute, 1971, 41-50.

Szekely, G. Developmental aspects of locomotion. In Herman, R., *et al.* (eds.) *Neural Control of Locomotion,* New York: Plenum Press, 1976, 735-757.

Taub, E. Motor behavior following deafferentation in the developing and motorically mature monkey. In Herman, R., *et al.* (eds.) *Neural Control of Movement,* New York: Plenum Press, 1976, 675-705.

Taub, E. Movement in non-human primates deprived of somato sensory feedback. In Wilmore, J., ed. *Exercise and Sports Science Review,* Santa Barbara, Cal.: Journal Publishing Affiliates, 1976, 335-374.

Victors, E. A. A cinematographic analysis of catching behavior of selected group of seven and nine year old boys. Unpublished doctoral dissertation, University of Wisconsin, Madison, 1961.

Whiting, H. T. A. Motor impairment – an overview. In Whiting, H. T. A., ed. *Concepts in Skill Learning,* London: Lepus Books, 1975, 91-108.

Whiting, H. T. A., & Hutt, J. W. R. The effect of personality and ability on speed of decision regarding directional aspects of bell-flight. *Journal of Motor Behavior,* 1974, *4,* 89-97.

3

Programs to Optimize
Infant Motor Development

MARCELLA V. RIDENOUR

Two major categories of programs today are designed to help develop infant motor skills. They differ primarily in the amount of
sensory and manual manipulation performed by a facilitator—usually a caretaker or parent. The first category, or No Programming
Plan, does not "prepractice" future motor skills, a facilitator will
not use passive, assisted movement, or specialized equipment to assist the infant's movement pattern and maintenance of posture.
The second type, or Programming Plan, on the other hand, encourages regular prepractice of future motor skills, using either
an infant motor curriculum, developmental exercises, or specialized equipment to assist with the performance of a motor skill.
Here we shall look at both motor development plans and critique
some of the techniques and equipment designed to accelerate the
motor development of infants.

The No Programming Plan for Infant Motor Development

The No Programming Plan is advocated by Emmi Pikler (1968)
of the National Methodological Institute for Infant Care and
Education, Budapest, Hungary. The institute withholds any form
of teaching or assistance while infants are learning posture and
motor skills. *Teaching* is defined by Pikler to be a systematic
practice of certain motor skills by holding or keeping the child in
a certain position, by adults, by equipment, or in anyway causing
him to make movements which he is not yet able to execute by

himself. Listed below are several motor enhancement guidelines
suggested by Pikler's No Programming Plan.

1. The infant is always lying on his back. He spends
    his waking time and sleeping time in this position
    until he is able to achieve another position by his
    own initiative without any assistance.
2. Toys are never placed in the infant's hand at any
    stage in development. All toys are placed near the
    infant on the floor. Toys are not hung above the
    infant's head. The infant must obtain the toys
    himself.
3. The infant who cannot yet sit upright is never
    placed in this position. The caretaker may not
    give the infant help to attain the sitting position.
    Infant seats or pillows are not used.
4. The infant who cannot independently attain stand-
    ing posture is not placed in the standing position.
5. A toddler who is able to walk only a few steps is
    not permitted to hold an adult's hand, even if he
    wants help to go for a longer walk.

The No Programming Plan is not varied for infants who are slow
in acquiring the normal postures and motor skills.

As part of the No Programming Plan, Pikler also advocates selecting infant clothes which will not restrict arm and leg movement. A wide sleeping sack is used during sleeping and resting
hours. The infant is never tucked or wrapped in blankets. The
baby wears pants as soon as he or she starts to roll on his side, to
encourage rolling. Hard-soled shoes are not worn until the child
walks independently—and only then when walking surfaces or
weather conditions make shoes necessary. During the daytime
the infant wears limited or no clothing.

Pikler bases her No Programming Plan of motor development
on observations with her own family, 10 years as a practicing
pediatrician, and her findings as a researcher at the Institute. Published reports by Pikler (1968) indicate the sequences of rolling,
creeping, sitting, standing, initial walking, and controlled walking

are similar to the acknowledged developmental schedules by Gesell (1941) and Illingworth (1960). One reported example of the superiority of her techniques involves successful creeping. The infants not only creep on the floor, but creep upstairs, on a ladder, and up and down a sloping terrain.

Programming Plan for Infant Motor Development

The Programming Plan is advocated by several Americans, primarily March Krottee, Professor of Physical Education, and Bonnie Prudden, authority on developmental fitness. A Programming Plan is also supported by a French physician, Dr. Janine Levy. These authorities have published books and reports describing appropriate activities for infants of varying chronological ages, from birth through 18 months (Prudden, 1964; Krottee, 1971; Levy, 1973). Most activities within their curricula involve practice of motor skills using either specialized equipment or manual manipulation of the infant's trunk, arms, or legs. Programming plans described in this chapter are the Prudden Infant Fitness Program, Levy Exercise Program, and Krottee Motor Development Curriculum.

The Prudden Infant Fitness Program

The Prudden program is written primarily for use by parents within the home (Prudden, 1964). It is a step-by-step, day-by-day program to enhance the child's fitness from birth to 6 years of age. The program begins with a series of 64 mother-infant activities for the first year. Bonnie Prudden provides a title and description of each activity as well as a photograph of a mother-infant pair performing it. The suggested program schedule is daily for about 15 minutes. All seven activities for the infant's first month require the mother to firmly hold and move the trunk, arms, or legs of the infant during the activity (Prudden, 1964). Two examples selected from the first seven exercises—bottoms up and chest stretch—are shown in Figures 3-1 and 3-2.

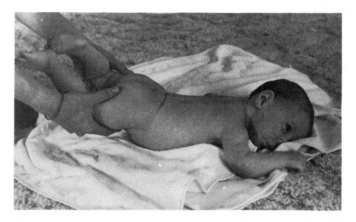

Figure 3-1. *Bottoms Up* requires the facilitator to slip her hands under the thigh and lift gently. It is recommended for the first two months.

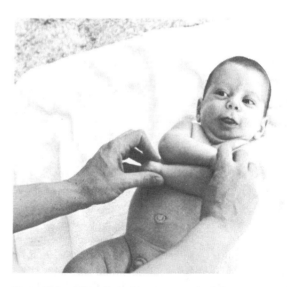

Figure 3-2. *Chest Stretch* encourages the infant to grasp the facilitator's forefingers while his arms are opened and extended. It is recommended for the first two months.

When the child is 3 months old, six new activities are introduced. These require the mother to hold firmly and move either the arms, legs, or trunk. An exception to this is encouraging the infant to freely kick after completing four sets of bicycle limb manipulations. Figure 3-3 illustrates The Tug, another suggested exercise for the 3-month-old infant. The activities for infants 4 through 12 months old include both activities that require complete movement manipulation of the child by the mother and activities permitting independent movement of the infant. Figure 3-4 illustrates one of the 51 activities suggested for this age group. Bonnie Prudden suggests the use of both the infant walker and baby bouncer. Her rationale for the infant walker is as follows: "This is a good way to keep a baby busy, right side up and out of the kitchen cabinets" (Prudden, 1964, p. 105). According

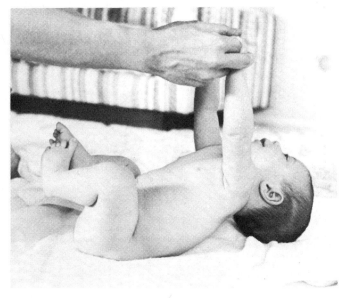

Figure 3-3. *The Tug* requires the infant to hold the facilitator's fingers while his upper back and shoulder are pulled to an arch position. It is recommended for the third month.

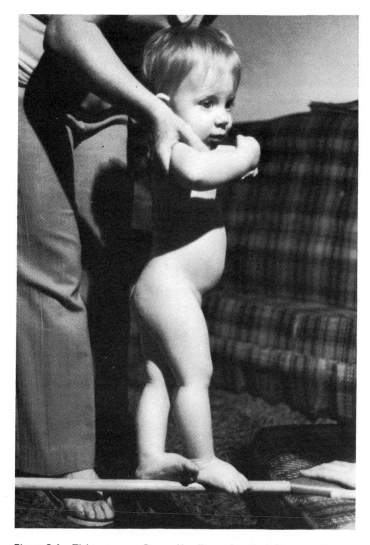

Figure 3-4. *Tightrope on a Broom Handle* requires the infant to walk on a horizontal broom handle with assistance from the facilitator. It is recommended for the 10 month old.

to Prudden, the best piece of infant apparatus is the jumper, since the infant is improving his posture and working his muscles while placed in the jumper. There is no appropriate age and/or developmental sequence suggested by Bonnie Prudden for initiating or discontinuing the use of the jumper or walker. This equipment, through physical and manual manipulation, permits the infant to perform prewalking and prejumping movements before he or she is able to walk and jump. The desirability of prewalking movements will be discussed in a later section of this chapter.

The Levy Exercise Program

The Levy exercise program is designed for infants up to 15 months old (Levy, 1973). The program emphasizes not manual manipulation of the infant but selected exercise based on his or her natural inclinations. The daily exercise program takes approximately 15 minutes. Overall, the program is divided into four phases:

1. Birth to 3 months: the period when movement education will be based on relaxing
2. 3 to 6 months: the phase of gymnastics preparation for sitting position.
3. 6 to 12 months: the phase of all-around movement, mastering the sitting position and preparation for standing
4. 9 to 15 months and beyond: the period of playing, mastering the standing position, and preparation for independence.

The following special equipment is needed for the Levy Program: tapered and cylindrical cushions, rag doll, beach ball, rods, baby walker cart with handle, hoop, stool, mirror, table, and toys.

In addition to 55 developmental exercises for infants, Levy makes the following suggestions to enhance motor development during the daily routine:

1. The infant's lying position is changed frequently: one side, flat on his back, or prone position. The prone

position is recommended for the first few weeks since
his hands are contacting the floor and he is less likely
to suck his thumb.

2. Shiny mobiles, rattles, and bright colored balls are suspended across the infant's crib.

3. During the daytime, the infant is flat on his tummy on
a floor mat. Toys should be around him (3 to 6
months).

4. The child may be placed in a semi-lying position in a
comfortable armchair. The semi-sitting position should
be limited to meal times (3 to 6 months).

5. The child is dressed in limited clothing (3 to 6 months).

6. The infant's use of the crib is limited to night time
only. The child should sleep on a foam rubber mat
during the day (6 months old).

7. A short stool is used to prepare and practice sitting.
The infant's feet should be flat on the floor, and initially the thigh should be held by the caretaker. Support should be removed gradually (5 to 7 months).

The 55 exercises generally involve optimizing the infant's
physical environment to facilitate independent performance of a
movement skill. Many of Levy's exercises do also require manual
manipulation of the limbs or trunk by the facilitator. Several of
these manipulative exercises are described as "relaxing exercises".
According to Levy, after general and local relaxation, the limbs
and body will loosen up and the child will sleep better and cry
less. Figures 3-5 through 3-9 illustrate five typical infant exercises in the Levy program.

The Krottee Curriculum

The Krottee curriculum is a series of interaction modules
(Krottee, 1971), each describing one activity for infants between
birth and 12 months old. The module describes the activity, response of the infant, method of evaluation, and appropriate reward for the infant. The reward is usually verbal praise of move-

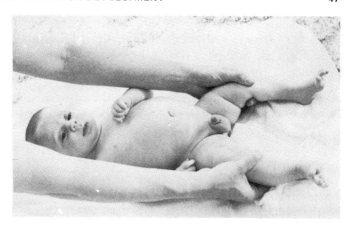

Figure 3-5. *Strengthening the Thighs* requires the facilitator to grasp the infant's knees and spread them apart. This exercise is recommended for the first 3 months of age.

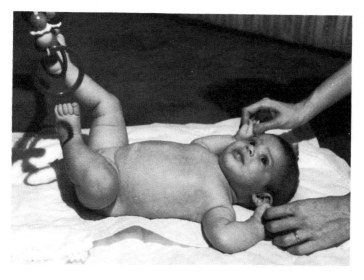

Figure 3-6. *Pedalling* encourages the infant to contact, grasp, and hold a suspended toy with his feet. This exercise is recommended for infants between 3 and 6 months old.

ment stimulation from the facilitator. The Krottee curriculum is extremely extensive and detailed. Over 100 activities are described, and the curriculum is designed for a child development professional rather than for use by the parent in the home (Krottee, 1971). The following five activities were selected to illustrate the Krottee curriculum:

The Stepping Game. This interaction module is intended for infants between birth and 1 month old. The infant is held by a facilitator in an upright position over a floor or table so the infant's feet are touching a flat surface (see Figure 3-10). The facilitator maintains facial contact and says, "step-step-step" as the infant's feet are lowered and placed on the surface. After 10 seconds of stepping, the infant is rewarded with a hug and a "good baby" reply.

The Mirror Game. This interaction module is intended for infants between 1 and 4 months old. The facilitator and infant are both sitting in front of the mirror. The facilitator says "see the baby?" If the infant notices his image and reaches for the mirror, the facilitator says "good baby." This module is assumed to be learned when the infant responds on 50 percent of the 10 trials presented daily for 3 days. Figure 3-11 illustrates the *Mirror Game.*

The Grab Grab Game. This interaction module is intended for infants between 1 and 4 months old. The infant is lying in a supine (back) position. The facilitator has an assortment of objects: paper, tin foil, sponge, plastic spoon, cloth, block, etc. The facilitator verbally rewards successful

grasps with a "good baby" reply. The procedure
is repeated with another object, alternating the
presentation to the opposite hand. Figure 3-12
illustrates the *Grab-Grab Game.*

Drop in the Bucket Game. This interaction module
is intended for infants between 8 and 12 months
old. The infant sits in front of a bucket. The
facilitator places a tennis ball in the infant's hands,
guides his hand into the bucket; then the infant
releases the ball. The infant is verbally rewarded
with a "big baby" reply for successful completion
of the guided sequence. The infant is encouraged
to get the ball out of the bucket at the end of the
sequence. Figure 3-13 illustrates the *Drop in the
Bucket Game.*

Summary and Issues

Advocates of both the non-programming and programming infant motor development enhancement environments present very
limited research to support their theories and programs (Prudden,
1964, Pikler, 1968; Levy, 1973; Krottee, 1971). A frequent illus-
tration of the Programming Plan is the frequent use of infant
walkers by parents desiring to accelerate the onset of independent
walking. Surveys by Ridenour have indicated 55 percent of the
parents with infants purchase and regularly use an infant walker
(Ridenour, 1973). Simpkiss and Raikes (1972) warn of potential
developmental abnormalities associated with infant walkers where
they observed exaggerated bilateral extensor thrust of the lower
limbs during weight bearing associated with poor balance. Hand
movements were clumsy and the acquisition of manipulative
skills was delayed; and when the infant was placed in sitting position, his propping mechanisms were poorly developed or delayed.
   Pontius (1975) expresses concern that the recent experimental

research, indicating the positive effects of early sensory stimulation, may be inaccurately generalized to daily repetitive exercising of the infant's stereotyped reflex movements, especially the stepping reflex. The stepping reflex is present in the newborn and its presence continues until the baby is approximately 11 months old. It may be the stepping reflex that accounts for the success of March Krottee's "stepping game" interaction module during the first months (Krottee, 1971). We are not yet certain of the purpose and function of the newborn reflexes (Pontius, 1973, 1975; Piaget, 1952; Zelazo et al., 1972, 1974). Some developmental psychologists encourage the exercise of newborn reflexive movements, such as the stepping and grasping reflexes Zelazo et al., 1972, 1974). The concept that the reflex movement precedes, and aids the development of, similar voluntary movements stems from interpretations of the observations by Piaget. The opposite view questions the role of reflexes such as the "stepping reflex" as a readiness and practice reflex because of the extremely unnatural position needed to elicit the reflex. The value and function of the "stepping reflex" is viewed as limited to serving survival in utero where it helps to bring the head into vertex position, the most propitious position for birth. (Langreder, 1949).

Limited experimental research is available to support either viewpoint. Experimental research by Zelazo et al. (1972) has indicated that systematic exercising of the stepping reflex (4 times daily in newborns from 1 week until 8 weeks in age) accelerates the normal development of walking. The experimental active-exercise group increased the frequency of walking, placing, and straightening responses during the 7-weeks experiment—as compared to the passive exercise group, no-exercise group, and 8-weeks control group. According to Zelazo, the results strongly confirm the hypothesis that walking among active-exercise infants seems to progress from a reflexive to an instrumental response. Follow-up data indicate that infants receiving active exercise walked sooner than infants in the other groups. The group means were 10.12 months for the active-exercise groups, 11.38 months for the passive-exercise group, 11.71 months for the no-exercise group, and 12.35 months for the control group. A similar study by Lagerspetz *et al.* (1971) examined the influence of a 3-week daily crawling exercise program on later creeping skill. The crawling exercises consisted of the experimenter helping the infant move forward by lifting his body and moving his head and arms alternately. The experimental group creeped significantly earlier, and transfer effects on other locomotor development were shown.

Severe criticism of both the Zelazo experimental design and the value of accelerated walking limit the interpretation and application of experimental results. For instance, at the natural age for walking, the soft spot on the head (anterior and posterior fontanel) is almost closed, but accelerated walking may expose infants who have incomplete closure of the soft spot to possible central nervous system injury. Also, relationships between infants with large leg muscle masses (as determined radiographically) and the early onset of walking indicate a minimum amount of muscle mass is needed to protect the long bones, and this may not be available for prematurely induced walking. Accelerated walking may interfere with the natural progressions of reflex development, especially if the infant spends less time than normal creeping (Gotts, 1972). One authority on the relationship between early motor development and later specific learning disabilities emphasizes the value of the total completion of the crawling-creeping sequence to facilitate complete neurological organization (Doman, 1974).

Other studies question the value of placing the infant in a mechanically or parentally assisted vertical position prior to the acquisition of independent sitting. A recent study by Gregg *et al.* (1976), comparing the visual tracking behavior of 48 neonates in both the horizontal and upright positions, indicates that the upright position had a negative effect on visual tracking performance. A study with similar results by Harper (1972) indicated that when mothers placed their infants under 3 months of age in an upright position the same infants, when 30 months old, were not so skillful as their prone or supine peers at manipulating objects. The results of these studies can be generalized to the importance of the prone and supine position for the infant rather than an assisted sitting or assisted standing position. Research by Brackbill *et al.* (1973) recommends the prone position over the supine position to reduce crying and movement, and encourage sleeping. No research data are available examining the effect of supine and prone positioning of an *awake* infant on later motor development.

The results of these studies indicate the confusion and contradiction in both the experimental and popular literature regarding stimulation of an infant's motor development by exercise or mechanical assistance. The American parenting environment involves many mechanical conveniences to assist with child care. Most parents have several of the following: playpen, walker, jumper, high chair, infant seat, or stroller. Yet excessive use of walking devices prior to independent walking may interfere with the quality of walking pattern (Simpkiss and Raikes, 1972), and the U.S. Consumer Product Safety Commission estimates that in the calendar year 1976 over 3919 infants received walker-related injuries. Most of these injuries were caused by the infant's tipping the walker over, poor structural design of the walker, or the infant's falling down steps. Since walker use has not been proven to improve walking performance and does present a safety hazard, parents should use the walker with caution because it may be both developmentally inappropriate and unsafe.

Until further and more conclusive research indicates the strengths and limitations of the non-programming and programming techniques for optimizing motor development, parents should avoid motor stimulation programs advertising excessive promises about the infant's future motor or intellectual performance. The popular books available do not provide enough information for parents to design a complete home infant exercise series of motor development curriculum. The preparation of teachers and facilitators for infants' motor development programs should include developmental kinesiology, biomechanics, motor develop-

ment, and developmental psychology.

Perhaps our emphasis should shift away from exercise classes for infants toward parenting classes to design the home and outdoor environment to facilitate the natural motor development of infants. Possibly future research may indicate a naturally changing floral garden with beautiful colors, shapes, textures, contours, surfaces, sounds, and moving objects (butterflies, birds, adults, other children, and other infants) as the optimal environment for an infant, providing there are adequate caretakers and facilitators available to assist and interact with the child—as requested by the infant himself through body movement and non-verbal communication.

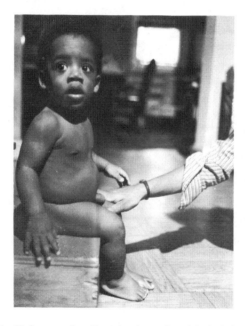

Figure 3-7. *Sitting on a Stool* is assisted exercise with the infant sitting on the stool and the facilitator only supporting the thigh. This exercise is recommended for infants between 6 and 12 months old

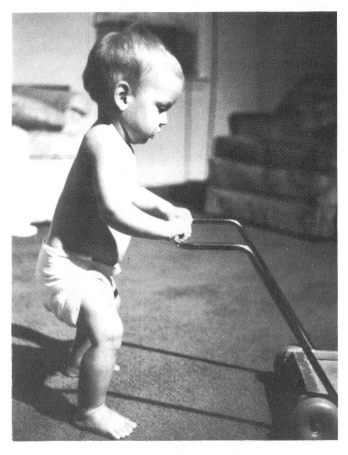

Figure 3-8. *The Baby-Walker* involves the use of a baby-cart-walker to assist the infant's prewalking and walking skills. This exercise is recommended for infants between 9 to 15 months old

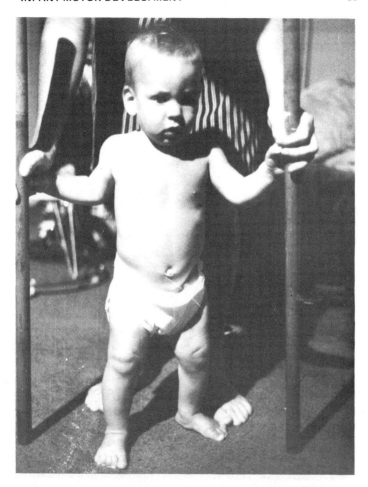

Figure 3-9. *The Rods* involves the use of two vertical rods supported by the facilitator, to assist the infant's pre-walking and walking skills. This exercise is recommended for infants between 9 and 15 months old

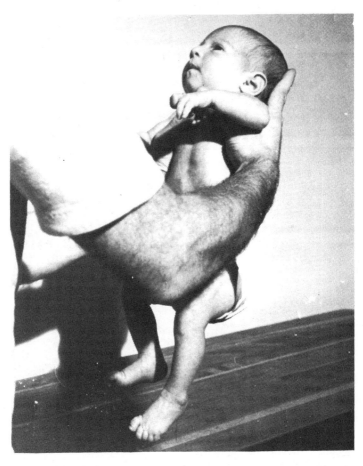

Figure 3-10. *The Stepping Game* encourages the infant to move his feet up and down while contacting a flat surface. It is recommended for infants during the first month.

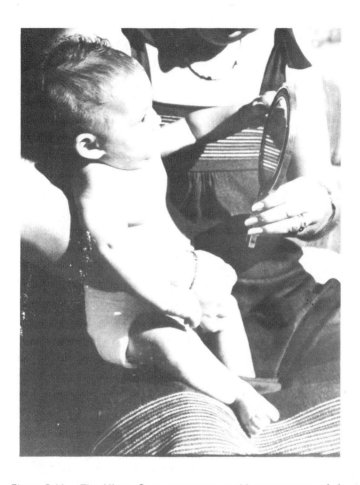

Figure 3-11. *The Mirror Game* encourages reaching movements of the infant. It is recommended for infants between 1 and 4 months old.

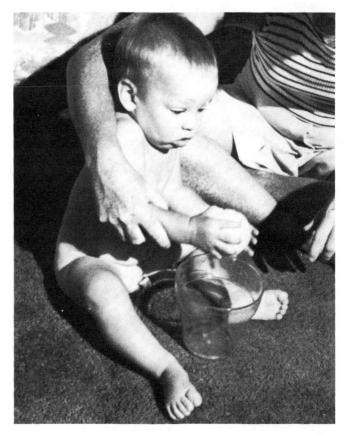

Figure 3-13. *Drop in the Bucket Game* encourages the infant to release the ball in a stationary target, a bucket. It is recommended for infants between 1 and 4 months old.

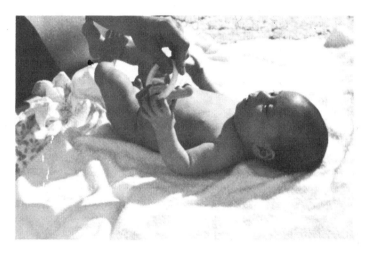

Figure 3-12. *The Grab Grab Game* encourages reaching movements of the infant. It is recommended for infants between 1 and 4 months old.

REFERENCES

Brackbill, Y., Douthitt, T., & West, H. Psychophysiologic effects in the neonate of prone versus supine placement. *The Journal of Pediatrics,* 1973, *82,* 82-84.

Cherry. R. Spare the exercise, spoil the child. *New York Times Magazine,* Feb. 9, 1975, 65-66, 69, 86.

Doman, G. *What to do About Your Brain-Injured Child.* Garden City, N.Y.: Doubleday, 1974.

Gessel, A. *Developmental Schedules.* New York: Psychological Corporation, 1941.

Gotts, E. E. Newborn walking. *Science,* 1972. *177,* 1057-1058.

Gregg, C. L., Haffner, G. M., & Korner, A. The relative efficacy of vestibular-proprioceptive stimulation and the upright position in enhancing visual pursuit in neonates. *Child Development,* 1976, *47,* 309-314.

Harper, L. Early maternal handling and preschool behavior of human children. *Developmental Psychobiology,* 1972, *5,* 1-5.

Illingsworth, R. S. *The Development of the Infant and Young Child, Normal and Abnormal.* London: Livingstone Ltd., 1960.

Jones, S. *Good Things for Babies.* Boston: Houghton Mifflin Company, 1976.

Krottee. M. The design of a curriculum for motor development in infants. Unpublished doctoral dissertation. University of Pittsburgh, 1971.

Langreder, W. Uber total reflexe und doren untrauterine bedeutung. *6 Gerburtsh, Gynak,* 1949, *131,* 237-252.

Lagerspetz, K., Nygard, M., & Stranduick, C. The effects of training in crawling on the motor and mental development of infants. *Scandinavian Journal of Psychology,* 1971, *12,* 192-197.

Levy, J. *The Baby Exercise Book,* New York: Random House, 1973.

Piaget, J. *The Origins of Intelligence.* New York: International University Press, 1952.

Pikler, E. Some contributions to the study of the gross motor development of children. *The Journal of Genetic Psychology,* 1968, *113,* 27-39.

Pontius, A. Neuro-ethics of walking in the newborn. *Perceptual and Motor Skills,* 1973, *37,* 235-245.

Pontius, A. New frontiers of ecological ethics, a balance between over and under control of outer and inner factors. *Experientia,* 1975, *31,* 263-264.

Prudden, B. *How to Keep Your Child Fit From Birth To Six.* New York: Harper & Row, 1964.

Ridenour, M. V. *Infant Walker Survey.* Unpublished report, Universtiy of Delaware 1973.

Simpkiss, M. V., & Raikes, A. J. Problems resulting from excessive use of baby-walkers and baby-bouncers. *Lancet,* 1972, *747,* 7753.

Zelazo, P., Kolb, S., & Zelazo, N. A. Newborn walking: a reply to Pontius. *Perceptual and Motor Skills,* 1974, *39,* 423-428.

Zelazo, P., Zelazo, N., & Kolb, S. Newborn walking. *Science,* 1972, *177,* 1058-1059.

Zelazo, P., Zelazo, N., & Kolb, S. Walking in newborns, *Science,* 1972, *176,* 314-375.

4

Stages in
Motor Development

MARY ANN ROBERTON

An intriguing notion in the study of motor behavior is the theory
that human movement develops in a predictable sequence of qualitative changes. These observable changes or "stages" are believed
to reflect a reconstruction of the nervous system; each stage represents the substitution of a new neural "program" for a previous
program. The sequence of stages is thought to be universal—all
people who show change in their motor behavior go through the
same stages in the same order.

Under this paradigm, the two tasks of the motor development
specialist are to identify (1) the stage sequences, and (2) the
mechanisms by which people change from stage to stage. In ex-
ploring the issue of motor stages, we can use these two tasks as a
chapter outline. We'll begin with the question of stage sequences—
first, as they are used in developmental psychology and, then, as
they are used in motor development.

Stages in Developmental Psychology

The concept of motor stages became popular in developmental
psychology due to Jean Piaget's cognitive research which began in
the 1920's and continues today. Previous to him, Sigmund Freud
(1930) adopted the stage notion to describe psychosexual development. Lawrence Kohlberg (1963), who studies moral reasoning, is the most recent developmentalist to use stage theory.

The best description of what stages are comes from Piagetian
theorists (Pinard & Laurendeau, 1969; Flavell & Wohlwill, 1969;
Inhelder, 1971). They use several characteristics to define stages.
The first is *hierarchical, qualitative change.* Something new occurs

in the behavior of the individual, a behavior never seen before, one which reflects the existence of a new mental "structure" and its concomitant functioning. The fact that the behavior is qualitatively different from preceding behaviors means it is not just an extension of those behaviors; more and more of a previous behavior never adds up to the new behavior. It is hierarchically different from the preceding behavior just as mammals are hierarchically different from reptiles although an outgrowth of them. In fact, stage theory sees development as an evolving of behavior, much as evolutionary theory sees organisms as evolving from one another through genetic mutation. Transitional periods connect the stages or evolutionary layers; but once the new level is reached, the behaviors or organisms are identifiably different; they are something "new."

Hierarchical incorporation of the preceding stage into the subsequent one is the second characteristic of stages. Each stage is different from, yet grows out of, and therefore incorporates, the preceding level. It does this by reorganizing or transforming the structures of that preceding level to form the new structures of the new level. This notion is called *hierarchical integration.*

Because stages evolve out of one another, they are also *intransitive.* Their ordering cannot be changed. Stage 1 must always precede stage 2, which must always precede stage 3. No individual could develop from stage 2 to 1 to 3. All individuals pass through this *universal stage sequence* in the same order, although they progress at their own rate and some people may never move through the entire sequence.

As stages evolve, they only gradually consolidate. Thus, various behaviors represented in the stage do not appear at once. Piagetians refer to this developmental lag between the behaviors of a stage as *horizontal décalage.* The consolidation process also allows behaviors from the preceding stage or the subsequent stage to mix with behaviors from the present stage; during these transitional periods each stage reveals the conclusion of a past stage or intimations of the next level to come.

One of the most important characteristics of a particular stage, however, is the unity of the internal structures and processes subserving that stage. This organic interconnection among stage processes can be called a *structural wholeness* and is reflected in all the task behaviors belonging to a stage.

Finally, the mechanism by which one moves through stages is known as the *equilibration process.* An imbalance between the mental structures and the environment is supposed to cause a behavioral action system to move out of its consolidated stage into a transition between stages and, then, into the next higher stage as reorganizing structures consolidate again. Overt behavior will reflect this equilibration process by showing periods of relative stability when in a consolidated stage and periods of instability when changing to a higher stage.

Stages in Motor Development

The word *stage* is often used in everyday language with no awareness of its theoretical meanings. For instance, a parent may speak of a child being in a "talkative stage," meaning simply a talkative time. This usage is atheoretical. The parent does not mean that talkativeness incorporates the characteristics defined for stages. The terms *point, phase, time,* or *mood* could all have been substituted for *stage* with no loss of meaning.

This atheoretical usage is also common in the motor development literature. For example, Halverson (1931) is well known for his *"stages"* of prehension, but he interchanged the word freely with *type* and *pattern* and seemed to attribute no theoretical significance to his word choice. More recently, Morris (1976) used the word *stage* to describe levels of difficulty within environmental factors that impinge upon children's movement. In his terminology, a child might be in a "stationary ball stage" of kicking. Clearly, this use of the word *stage* refers to the environment (the ball), whereas stage theory refers to the child's movement in reference to that ball and to the hypothetical structures underlying the movement. Again, Morris was using *stage* atheoretically. He could have substituted any number of words to mean "levels of difficulty."

Other motor development researchers, however, have consciously accepted the theory behind the term *stage,* although they may not have understood it in the fullness of Piagetian criteria. For instance, Gesell defined stages as a "series of postural transformations" (1946, p. 302). Ames called them a "uniform sequence of . . . behavior patterns" (1937, p. 423). In 1931, John E. Anderson stressed the orderliness of motor development "in which different types of response unfold at successive stages" (p. v). Seefeldt, Reuschlein, & Vogel (1972) defined stages as the "commonality of [body] segmental relationships between performers" (p. 9). These researchers all chose the term *stages* purposely to stress the universal, sequential, hierarchical appearance of the movements they had observed. In addition, belief in the intransitivity of that hierarchy was stated or implied in the motor development research of Burnside (1927), Ames (1937, 1966), Shirley (1931), Gesell (1946), and Wild (1937).

Even the concept of equilibration was expressed by Gesell (1946) as he studied what he called the "reciprocal interweaving" of flexion and extension across the stages of prone behavior. He saw development as a self-regulated, oscillating spiral through these stages, a spiral which resulted in a "state of unstable and shifting equilibrium" (p. 289). Thus, the idea of stages is in no sense borrowed from cognitive psychology. It has a long history as a developmental theory in the study of motor behavior.

One important motor development theorist, McGraw, (1935, 1943), however, purposely refused to use the word *stage.* She opted, instead, to describe "phases" in infant motor development. Yet, of all motor development theorists, McGraw was the strongest advocate for the notion of qualitative change. She wrote, "[Development is] the *emergence* of something new—a way of behaving in which that particular individual has never behaved before" (McGraw, 1975, p. 301). Modern theorists would recognize her definition as synonymous with the stage criterion of hierarchical, qualitative change. McGraw's avoidance of the word *stage* seems based on the belief that stages implied saltatory changes in behavior, abrupt jumps from one way of acting to the next.[1] This notion is an unnecessary corollary of stage theory and has been

---

[1] McGraw, M. Personal communication, Summer, 1976.

disclaimed by stage theorists (Flavell & Wohlwill, 1969; Pinard & Laurendeau, 1969; Wohlwill, 1973). Piaget and Kohlberg, for instance, stress the gradual transition that takes place during the consolidation process (Wohlwill, 1973; Turiel, 1969). The belief that stages mean abrupt change in behavior is a common misconception about this developmental theory.

Testing Motor Stages

Being a developmental theory, the notion of motor stages is open to testing. Motor stages should conform to the criteria cited earlier for all developmental stages—yet no one has ever measured proposed motor stages against these criteria. Early motor development researchers seemed to accept stages as a developmental "given" rather than as a theory to be tested. They expected to find stages and so they did!

The most testable aspects of stage theory are the concepts of a universal stage sequence and intransitivity. To test these two concepts fully, many individuals must be followed longitudinally to see if they actually go through each of the hypothesized stages. Since these concepts assume the position of a "law" in developmental theory, the most rigorous test would be an idiographic one, that is, a case-by-case test. If one finds a "negative case"—someone who does not move through the stages in the order hypothesized—then the law is refuted. After such refutation, some theorists might still wish to claim that stages were a developmental "trend" which most people tended to show, but they could not claim stages were a developmental law which applied universally to all people.

Most of the studies which "discovered" stages for various motor tasks were not designed to test either the universality or the intransitivity of the sequences they proposed. The studies usually compared people of different ages rather than following the same people as they aged. Thus, the stages were always from a composite of subjects, only some or none of whom had actually been observed to pass through *all* the stages in the order hypothesized. Shirley (1931) and Ames (1937) were among the few early researchers to offer some longitudinal support for their claim that all subjects went through all stages. Shirley designed her five major stages of walking so infants might shift the order of substages within a stage as they developed but not the order of the major stages. Ames reported that of 5 infants on whom she had full data, 4 showed all 14 of her prone progression stages, one showed 13 of the 14. Of a total of 20 infants observed, however, only 8 showed all 14 stages; 11 skipped 1 or 2 stages; and 1 skipped more than 2 stages. These stage "skips" she attributed to incomplete data rather than to the children. Gesell (1946) felt Ames' figures gave support to the stage concept, although by idiographic criteria they do not.

The only study actually designed to test the universality and intransitivity of a set of motor stages was one by Roberton (1977c). She developed a two-phase research approach which first examined children's movement across trials at one point in time. Stage theory predicts that if people go through stages in learning a motor task, they should look rather stable or consistent in their movement during the time they are in a particular stage. If they are observed across trials at this time, they should consistently use the same movements from trial to trial. If they vary at all, they should vary to the movements of either the stage immediately lower or the one immediately higher—that is, to the adjacent stage. Such variation would indicate they were in transition to the next stage above them, or that they were showing vestiges of the stage they had just left. In all cases, however, they would exhibit movements characteristic only of adjacent stages in the hypothesized stage ordering. The subjects would also show a modal stage frequently enough that they could be identified as being in a consolidated stage.

Using this across-trials approach, Roberton studied hypothesized stages of the forceful overarm throw. She independently classified the movements observed in each of 10 trials of throwing for 73 first-grade children. Their movement had been recorded on 16mm film, which allowed repeated study of simultaneous side and rear views. Roberton found that all the children varied only to adjacent categories of arm action in the throw and that each child had at least half his trials classified into the same category. This was the criterion she had established for identifying a child as being in a stage. Her results agreed with the notions of a universal, intransitive stage sequence. Stage categories for trunk (pelvic-spinal) action in the throw, however, were not similarly supported. One child of the 73 had less than 5 trials in 1 stage category, making the concept of stage questionable. Several children also skipped to non adjacent categories across the 10 trials.

In the second phase of the study, Roberton refilmed the same children over 3 years. She is now studying the longitudinal data to see if the stage categories which survived the across-trial scrutiny will still prove to be universal and intransitive over time. A preliminary report of this longitudinal phase suggested that some of the stages may, in fact, prove to have these two characteristics (Roberton, 1977b).

At this point, however, the motor development literature contains minimal support for the notion of a sequence of motor stages common to all people who transverse it in the same order. Shirley's (1931) major stages of walking seemed intransitive, but it is not clear that they are universal. Ames' (1937) stages were not supported by her data as either intransitive or universal. Roberton (1977c) may have support for certain parts of the overarm throw but not for the entire throw. None of the other "stages" proposed in the literature offered any evidence for their intransitivity or universality. Clearly, more research is needed on this question. Indeed, no one has even begun to examine proposed motor stages in light of other stage criteria. We will look at the criterion of structural wholeness in the next section as a first attempt in this area.

Conceptualizing Motor Stages

The stages that have been proposed in the motor development literature vary in concept. Shirley's (1931) stages of locomotion are mainly between-task stages. "Creep" is a different task than "sit alone momentarily," which differs again from "walk alone" (see Table 4-1). Most other proposed stages (see, for example, Seefeldt *et al.*, 1972; Wickstrom, 1977) have taken one task, such as creeping, and described the development of movements from the first time the task is attempted until it is accomplished in an adult manner (see Table 4-2). These stages have been termed *intra-task stages* (Halverson, *et al.*, 1973) or *intra-skill stages* (Seefeldt *et al.*, 1972). A third stage type now has appeared with Roberton's (1977c) proposal for stages within "components" of a task. Her stages deal with the development of body areas, such as leg action or arm action, within the task (see Table 4-3). This approach has also been adopted by Roberton & Halverson (1977).

Table 4-1. Stages in Locomotor Development

Chin up
Chest up
Stepping
Sit on lap
Sit alone momentarily
Knee push or swim
Rolling
Stand with help
Sit alone 1 minute
Some progress on stomach
Scoot backward
Stand holding to furniture
Creep
Walk when led
Pull to stand
Stand alone
Walk alone

SOURCE: Shirley, M. *The First Two Years, A Study of Twenty-Five Babies.* The University of Minnesota Press, 1931.

Of these three approaches, which makes the most sense according to stage theory? The stage criterion known as *structural wholeness* is important here. The structural wholeness of a stage

Table 4-2. Stages in Overarm Throwing

Stage 1. Motion is essentially posterior-anterior in direction, feet remain fixed, little or no trunk rotation, force of movement comes from hip flexion, shoulder protraction, and elbow extension.

Stage 2. Feet remain fixed, increased rotation noted in hips and spine, force is directed more toward a transverse plane than in stage 1, rotation is about an imaginary vertical axis.

Stage 3. Primary change from stage two is that the movement is ipsilateral; i.e., the foot on the same side as the throwing arm strides in the direction of the throw. The trunk rotation *may be* decreased in relation to stage 2, but the hip flexion is increased.

Stage 4. The movement is contralateral; i.e., this stage shows opposition of movement in that the foot opposite the throwing arm strides forward in the "wind-up" phase, thus allowing a greater range of motion. The time over which the forces can act is thus greatly increased.

SOURCE: Seefeldt, V., Reuschlein, S. and Vogel, P. Sequencing motor skills within the physical education curriculum. Paper presented to the National Convention of the American Association for Health, Physical Education, and Recreation, 1972; after Wild, M. The behavior pattern of throwing and some observations concerning its course of development in children. Unpublished doctoral dissertation, University of Wisconsin-Madison, 1937.

causes a person to attack all related tasks in the same way. Thus, the stage concept is really a multiple task notion, a multivariate notion (Wohlwill, 1973). For instance, a child in "stage 1" should show that stage in the movements he uses for throwing *and* striking. In this vein, there would be stages of locomotion rather than stages of hopping. A stage should be seen in several tasks at once, giving it horizontal as well as vertical (hierarchical) structure. Using this criterion, none of the three approaches currently in the motor development literature would qualify as stages even if they met the criteria of universality and intransitivity. For instance, Shirley's "stages" (Table 4-1) are primarily an age ordering of tasks. They are qualitatively different

Table 4-3. Trunk Action (Pelvic-Spinal) Stages in the Overarm Throw

      A. Common pelvic-spinal channel
           1. No trunk action
           2. Extension and/or flexion of the trunk
           3. Spinal rotation with the pelvis stationary
                or spinal-then-pelvic rotation
           4. Block rotation of the trunk

Then, either

B. Overarm channel	C. Sidearm channel
5. Block rotation plus lateral flexion of the trunk	5. Differentiated rotation
6. Differentiated rotation plus lateral flexion of the trunk	

SOURCE: Roberton, M. A. Stability of stage categorizations across trials: Implications for the "stage theory" of overarm throw development. *Journal of Human Movement Studies*, 1977,*3*, 49-59.

and predictable, but there "is no more reason to label each of these responses as a 'stage' than there is, for example, to apply that term to places on the itinerary of a bus line" (Wohlwill, 1973, p. 193). This does not mean, however, that Shirley has not identified a legitimate developmental sequence—although, as mentioned earlier, it may not be universal.

One of the dangers in calling age-ordered tasks "stages" can be seen in the Delacato (1963) perceptual-motor training controversy. Considering all tasks which develop before other tasks *prerequisites* for those subsequent tasks (as previous stages are prerequisites to subsequent stages) leads to strange conclusions. Because losing one's first tooth developmentally precedes driving a car, is it legitimate to say the former is prerequisite to the latter? Yet, this is the reasoning used by Delacato when he said that *because* cross-pattern creeping precedes reading, it is therefore prerequisite to reading. Furthermore, since it is prerequisite to reading, practice in cross-pattern creeping will help poor readers improve their reading! Clearly, this thinking represents a misapplication of stage theory.

To make the question of Shirley's "stages" more complex, it is quite possible that some of her stages *are* prerequisite to others. For example, "chin up" and "chest up" are prerequisite to "sit alone 1 minute," but "stand holding to furniture" would not seem prerequisite to "creep." What we need is a revamping of most infant stage sequences to distinguish those parts which are the ordering of tasks and those parts which are orderings within tasks. Shirley actually began this procedure by dividing her stages into first to fifth "order skills."

Within-task or intra-task orderings are the most frequent type of stage encountered in motor development (see Table 4-2). Again, because they are limited to one task, they do not generalize broadly enough to have the breadth implied by structural wholeness; however, they can be legitimate developmental sequences. Wohlwill (1973) has suggested that levels within such sequences be called *steps.* These steps can also be intransitive and universal.

Roberton (1977*b*) has indicated an additional problem with most of the intra-task stages currently in the motor development literature. All of them depict total body changes from one level or step to the next. They predict what the feet, the head, the arms, etc., will look like, at a given level. This approach implies that everyone who has ever learned to throw a ball, for instance, has looked the same way as they learned. Observers trying to classify people into these stages know that everyone does not look exactly the same. Perhaps the trunk action is the same as described in the stage, but the feet don't match, or the arm action varies. To use these total-body stages, the observer inevitably weighted one or more components of the configuration more than others: if the feet didn't fit the stage description, but the trunk action did, he'd probably classify the person according to trunk action.

Data reported by Roberton (1977*b*) indicated that for the overarm throw, development did not take place in lock-step, total-body changes but, rather, that certain movements or components of the body action changed while others did not. Table 4-4 indicates her results for three components of the throw. It is clear that not all parts of the body showed synchronous development. Of 54 children filmed yearly for 3 years, only 6 percent showed change in both their humeral action and their trunk action. Only 7 percent showed change in both their humeral action and their relative length of stride. Some children showed change in humeral action but not the other component; some showed change in the other component but not humeral action.

Table 4-4. Relationship Between Humeral Development and Development in Two Other Components of the Overarm Throw

Component				
Humerus	Trunk Action		Relative Length of Stride	
	Changed	Did Not Change	Changed	Did Not Change
Changed	6%	30%	7%	28%
Did not change	19%	46%	17%	48%

Note: N=54.

SOURCE: Roberton, M. A. Stability of stage categorizations in motor development. Paper presented to the annual convention of the North American Society for the Psychology of Sport and Physical Activity. Ithaca, N.Y., 1977.

Roberton cited this data as evidence for the invalidity of the intra-task stages presently in the literature and as support for her "component model of intra-task motor development" (Roberton, 1977c). She felt that if there were stages of motor task development, perhaps these stages occurred only in the components rather than in the total body configuration. Thus, in throwing, a child might move ahead a stage in his trunk action while retaining the same stage of arm action. Another child might keep his trunk action stage but move ahead in his arm action. Two children moving through the same stages in each component would show a different combination of those stages at any one time. Few people would ever be at the same point in all their component stages at the same time, so few people would look exactly the same as they learned to throw a ball. Yet they would have gone through the same stages of development (see Figure 4-1).

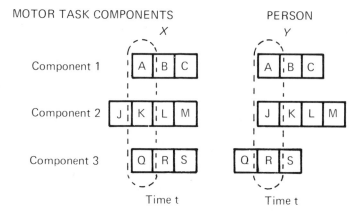

Figure 4-1. Model for the juxtaposition of intra-task motor components. Persons X and Y have the same intratask components with the same stages of development within each component; however, at time t person X shows the stages A, K, Q across components while person Y shows A, J, R. Component 2 has developed more rapidly in person X; component 3 more rapidly in person Y. From Roberton, M. A. Stability of stage categorizations across trials: Implications for the "stage theory" of overarm throw development. *Journal of Human Movement Studies,* 1977, *3,* 49-59.

Roberton's new model of intra-task development attempts to conceptualize the orderly patterns of motor development stressed by motor development researchers, yet still allow the rich individual differences which any developmental theory needs to recognize. The strength of the model is that it is not tied to stage theory *per se* and would apply even if stages were shown not to exist. Since Roberton has called the levels within her proposed developmental sequences *intra-task stages*, however, it should be pointed out that these "stages" also lack the broadness needed for the concept. To avoid semantic confusion, a better word choice would again be *steps*. These steps could well be intransitive and universal, as Roberton (1977*c*) suggested.

It would seem, then, that none of the three forms of "stages" presently described in the motor development literature fulfill the structural wholeness criterion for developmental stages. To clarify the semantic confusion, intra-task sequences could be said to contain *steps* rather than *stages*. Between-task orderings should simply be called *task sequences*. The notion of *stage* could then be reserved for movement commonalities that are observed in the way an individual approaches several motor tasks at the same point in time. Atheoretical usage of the word stage might also be lessened through this jargon clarification.

Questions about General Stages

Limiting the word *stage* in this way would not lessen the importance of identifying developmental sequences between and within tasks. It would, however, open new questions for research scrutiny. If these across-task, general motor stages exist, what is their implication for the generality-specificity argument once prevalent in motor learning literature? Clearly, if a person in a given stage approaches several tasks in the same way, there should be generality in his or her learning of those tasks. Evidence for this generality is lacking in studies using product score variables. Would it be found if one focused on the movements being used (Seefeldt *et al.*, 1972)? If motor stages exist, is there a horizontal décalage among the tasks represented in the stage? That is, does the stage show up asynchronously across tasks, or would it appear in all tasks simultaneously? If motor stages exist, do certain steps from within-task sequences belong in one motor stage while other steps belong in a higher stage? Finally, if motor stages exist only in components of the movements, as Roberton (1977c) proposed, does one see the same component stage in several tasks at the same point in time? This new notion of across-task, general motor stages invites many questions for future research.

Stages or Steps as Dependent Variables

So far, this discussion has dealt solely with the first task of the motor development specialist under the stage paradigm—identifying valid stage sequences. If this task is ever successfully accomplished, then the second task would be to identify the *mechanisms* of stage change. In cognitive development, for example, Pascual-Leone (1970) has attempted to explain movement through stages in terms of information-processing capacity. Does his cognitive paradigm apply to movement through motor stages? Todor (1975) and Thomas (Thomas & Bender, 1976) have begun to investigate this question, although a relationship between cognitive stages and motor stages has not yet been established. Could another information-processing model apply—one which showed concomitant changes in the way information was handled by the nervous system for each motor stage observed? In a more traditional vein, what changes in the environment accompany motor stage changes? What physiological changes accompany them?

To answer these questions, the general motor stage or the step in an intra-task sequence will become the dependent variable. Manipulations of the environment or of the information the subject receives will allow us to see if the stage or step is changed. In some sense, much of the completed motor development research could be replicated using stages or steps as dependent variables instead of the product scores previously used. For instance, we know boys throw farther than girls, but do they throw using qualitatively more advanced movements? Will more boys be found at higher steps than girls of the same age? We also know that children throw farther as they increase in age, but do they show concomitant intra-task step development? Roberton (1977b) has presented some startling preliminary data on throwing which show almost half of 54 children *not* improving in several important throwing components from kindergarten through second grade. Since these children were receiving physical education twice weekly, this result also questions the effect of instruction and practice on motor steps and stages. In addition, we could ask, do child-rearing practices affect motor stage change? Could training in the observation of motor stages help teachers improve their teaching (Roberton, 1977a) and parents improve their parenting? Clearly, with so many questions unanswered, the fun in motor stage research has just begun!

The Motor Stage Issue

What, then, is the status of the issue of motor stages? Although the theory has been around for a long while, relatively little research has explored the question. What little there is seems inconclusive. A stage definition more in line with the definition proposed for developmental stages in other action systems might help clarify the issue and highlight questions needing research. Until that research is carried out, however, the issue of motor stages will remain only an interesting speculation.

REFERENCES

Ames, L. Individuality of motor development. *Journal of the American Physical Therapy Association,* 1966, *46,* 121-127.

Ames, L. The sequential patterning of prone progression in the human infant. *Genetic Psychology Monographs,* 1937, *19,* 409-460.

Anderson, J. Foreword to M. Shirley, *The First Two Years, A Study of Twenty-Five Babies.* Minneapolis: The University of Minnesota Press, 1931.

Burnside, L. Coordination in the locomotion of infants. *Genetic Psychology Monographs,* 1927, *2,* 283-372.

Delacato, C. *The Diagnosis and Treatment of Speech and Reading Problems.* Springfield, Ill.: Thomas, 1963.

Flavell, J., & Wohlwill, J. Formal and functional aspects of cognitive development. In Elkind, D., & Flavell, J., eds. *Studies in Cognitive Development.* New York: Oxford University Press, 1969.

Freud, S. *Three Contributions to the Theory of Sex.* New York: Nervous and Mental Disease Publishing Co., 1930.

Gesell, A. The ontogenesis of infant behavior. In Carmichael, L., ed. *Manual of Child Psychology.* New York: Wiley, 1946.

Halverson, H. An experimental study of prehension in infants by means of systematic cinema records. *Genetic Psychology Monographs,* 1931, *10,* 107-286.

Halverson, L., Roberton, M. A., & Harper, C. Current research in motor development. *Journal of Research and Development in Education,* 1973, *6,* 56-70.

Inhelder, B. Criteria of the stages of mental development. In Tanner, J., and Inhelder, B., eds. *Discussions on Child Development.* New York: International Universities Press, 1971.

Kohlberg, L. The development of children's orientations toward a moral order. I. Sequence in the development of moral thought. *Vita Humana,* 1963, *6,* 11-33.

McGraw, M. *Growth, A Study of Johnny and Jimmy.* New York: Arno Press Reprint of the 1935 edition, 1975.

McGraw, M. *The Neuromuscular Maturation of the Human Infant.* New York: Hafner Reprint of the 1943 edition, 1963.

Morris, G. S. *How to Change the Games Children Play.* Minneapolis: Burgess, 1976.

Pascual-Leone, J. A mathematical model for the transition rule in Piaget's developmental stages. *Acta Psychologica,* 1970, *32,* 301-345.

Piaget, J. The attainment of invariants and reversible operations in the development of thinking. In Campbell, S., ed. *Piaget Sampler.* New York: Wiley, 1976.

Pinard, A., & Laurendeau, M. "Stage" in Piaget's cognitive-developmental theory: Exegesis of a concept. In Elkind, D., & Flavell, J., eds., *Studies in Cognitive Development.* New York: Oxford University Press, 1969.

Roberton, M. A. Motor stages: Heuristic model for research and teaching. Paper presented to the National Convention of the National Associations for Physical Education for College Men and Women, Orlando, Fla., 1977 (*a*).

Roberton, M. A. Stability of stage categorizations across trials: Implications for the "stage theory" of overarm throw development. *Journal of Human Movement Studies,* 1977, *3,* 49-59 (*c*).

Roberton, M. A. Stability of stage categorizations in motor development. Paper presented to the annual convention of the North American Society for the Psychology of Sport and Physical Activity, Ithaca, N.Y., 1977 (*b*).

Roberton, M. A., & Halverson, L. The developing child—His changing movement. In Logsdon, B., ed. *The Child in Physical Education - A Focus on the Teaching Process.* Philadelphia: Lea & Febiger, 1977.

Seefeldt, V., Reuschlein, S., & Vogel, P. Sequencing motor skills within the physical education curriculum. Paper presented to the National Convention of the American Association for Health, Physical Education, and Recreation, 1972.

Shirley, M. *The First Two Years, A Study of Twenty-Five Babies.* Minneapolis: The University of Minnesota Press, 1931.

Thomas, J., & Bender, P. A developmental explanation for children's motor behavior: A neo-Piagetian interpretation. In Christina, R., & Landers, D., eds. *Psychology of Motor Behavior and Sport—1976,* vol. II. Proceedings of the annual conference of the North American Society for the Psychology of Sport and Physical Activity, Austin, Tex., 1976.

Tudor, J. Age differences in integration of components of a motor task. *Perceptual and Motor Skills,* 1975, *41,* 211-215.

Turiel, E. Developmental processes in the child's moral thinking. In Mussen, P., Langer, J., & Covington, M., eds. *Trends and Issues in Developmental Psychology.* New York: Holt, Rinehart & Winston, 1969.

Wickstrom, R. *Fundamental Motor Patterns.* Philadelphia: Lea & Febiger, 1977.

Wild, M. The behavior pattern of throwing and some observations concerning its course of development in children. Unpublished doctoral dissertation, University of Wisconsin-Madison, 1937. (For a less complete version see *Research Quarterly,* 1938, *9,* 20-24.)

Wohlwill, J. *The Study of Behavioral Development.* New York: Academic Press, 1973.

5

Sex-Role Expectations
and Motor Behavior
of the Young Child

JACQUELINE HERKOWITZ

Sex-role expectations profoundly influence the movement behavior of young children. We can begin to understand their influence first by documenting the discrepancies in performance which exist between boys and girls on common motor tasks, and then by evaluating the extent to which these discrepancies can be explained by the anatomical and physiological differences between the sexes.

Performance Differences on Motor Tasks

Generally speaking, the running, throwing, jumping, hopping, kicking, catching, and striking performances of both boys and girls continue to improve to adolescence, with boys performing better than girls in almost all skill categories at almost all ages. Boys generally continue to improve through their late teens. Girls' performances, on the other hand, frequently level òr even drop off after 12 or 13 years of age.

Running. Data on the running of 30- to 50-yard sprints (American Association of Health, Physical Education, and Recreation, 1965; Espenschade, 1960; Glassow & Kruse, 1960; Jenkins, 1930; Keogh, 1965; Seils, 1951) depict consistent year-to-year improvements in running speed for both boys and girls, 5 to 11 years of age. Each year both sexes run approximately 1 foot per second faster, and boys tend to run approximately 1/3 foot per second faster than girls. From 11 to 17 years, girls' performances level and eventually drop off while those of boys continue to improve, though at a slower rate.

Throwing. Boys between 5 and 17 years old throw farther than girls of the same age, and discrepancies between the boys' and girls' performances increase with age. The difference is approximately 5 feet at 5 years, 25 feet at 8 years, and over 30 feet at 11 years (American Association for Health, Physical Education, and Recreation, 1965; Espenschade, 1960; Jenkins, 1930; Jones, 1951; Keogh, 1965; Seils, 1951).

Studies of throwing accuracy and the development of efficient overarm throwing patterns illustrate similar trends. Keogh (1965) found that the throwing accuracy of 7-, 8-, and 9-year-old children increases with increasing age and that boys perform more accurately than girls at all three age levels. Cinematographic studies of the development of overarm throwing indicate that boys and girls both demonstrate increasingly more efficient throwing patterns as they grow from 2 to 6½. Boys, however, demonstrate efficient throwing patterns earlier than do girls (Wild, 1938; Halverson & Roberton, 1966).

Jumping. As they grow from 5 to 11 years of age, children can jump about 4 inches more each year. Boys jump 1 to 4 inches farther than girls do, depending on the year. Boys between 12 and 17 years continue to improve their long jump in the same fashion, while girls' performances at these ages level off (American Association for Health, Physical Education, and Recreation, 1965; Espenschade, 1960; Glassow & Kruse, 1960; Jenkins, 1930; Keogh, 1965; Latchaw, 1954; Seils, 1951).

The jump and reach performances of 7- through 11-year-olds also improve with increasing age. Though no sex differences in performance are apparent at 7, boys are jumping approximately 1 to 2 inches higher than girls at 8, 9, 10, and 11 (Johnson, 1962).

Hopping. When Jenkins (1930) and Keogh (1965) asked 5- through 11-year-olds to hop 50 feet as fast as possible, they found that both boys and girls cut their time considerably (3 seconds) between 5 and 6 years of age, and then more gradually until they were 11 years old. Girls performed better than boys at all ages, with little discrepancy between the sexes at 5, 6, 10, and 11 years, and a greater discrepancy between the sexes at 7, 8, and 9 years.

Kicking. Only limited information exists regarding the kicking performances of children. The data available indicate that a general trend to improve exists for both sexes with increasing age, and that at all ages boys perform better than do girls. For 5-, 6- and 7-year-old boys and girls, respectively, Jenkins (1930) found that their average soccer kicks were 11.5 feet and 8.0 feet, 18.4 feet and 10.1 feet, 25.4 feet and 15.0 feet. Boys and girls in grades 1 through 6, performing the soccer punt for distance (Hanson, 1965) and kicking for accuracy (Johnson, 1962) improved with each grade level. Boys kicked better than girls at all grade levels, with performance discrepancies between the sexes growing larger in successive grades.

Catching. Hoadley's study (1941) of the catching ability of 250 elementary school children, when three different sized balls were used, demonstrated that boys and girls improve in the ability to catch large and small balls in grades 1 through 4. Boys were able to catch a small ball better than girls in grades 2, 3, and 4.

Striking. A variety of diverse striking tasks has been examined in children 5 through 10 years of age (e.g., volleyball service, strikes at balls swung over a plate on a string). Generally, boys have been found the better "strikers," with both sexes performing better each year (Hanson, 1965; Johnson, 1962; Seils, 1951).

Structural and Anatomical Differences

Discrepancies in motor performance between the sexes can be explained, to some extent, by structural and physiological differences.

Height and Weight. From birth to approximately 12 years of age, boys tend to be slightly taller than girls. From approximately 12 to 14 years, this trend reverses itself, and then between 14 and 18 years boys regain the stature advantage, which they keep through adulthood. Boys tend to be slightly heavier than girls from birth through 4 years. There are virtually no differences in the weight of boys and girls between the ages of 4 and 11. However, between 11 and 15, girls are generally heavier than boys; and at approximately 15 years, this trend reverses itself. Boys then become considerably heavier than girls and remain so in adulthood (Tanner, Whitehouse, & Takaishi, 1966).

The *rate* of height and weight growth in both boys and girls decreases sharply between birth and 2 years of age. During the elementary school years the rate of gain in weight slowly decreases while the rate of gain in height slowly increases. Girls reach their adolescent height and weight spurts at approximately 12 and 12½ years, respectively. Boys reach these same spurts at approximately 14 and 14½ years respectively (Tanner, Whitehouse, & Takaishi, 1966).

The height and weight growth characteristics of boys and girls in elementary school provides little explanation for their differences in physical skills. The earlier maturation rate of girls—and their actual height and weight advantage between 12 and 14, and 11 and 15, years respectively—should serve to decrease performance differences between the sexes at those times. In fact, however, the height and weight advantage of girls during these periods does not appear to influence performance significantly. The height and weight advantages enjoyed by boys from approximately 14 and 15 years, respectively, would help to explain their consistently better performances during this age period. But what about the fact that peak growth rate in adolescence is approximately 2 years earlier for girls than for boys? The period of relative growth stability prior to adolescence should first favor the physical performances of boys, and then those of girls. Once again, however, this growth factor does not seem to influence performance trends one way or another.

Body Proportions. Boys and girls between 2 and 6 years old show few differences in the proportional growth of their body segments which would account for motor performance differences. Girls maintain a relatively longer leg length in comparison to sitting height than do boys. But they maintain the same ratio of shoulder width to pelvic breadth, although the actual measurements for males are slightly larger than those for females (Sinclair, 1973).

From 7 to 12 years, the limbs continue to grow more than the trunk, particularly in boys. Another sex difference that emerges after 6 years is the relationship of pelvic breadth to shoulder width (Sinclair, 1973). Gain in shoulder width is approximately the same for both sexes for 6- to 10-year-olds, but girls gain more in hip width. After 10, boys increase considerably more in shoulder width than girls do. The longer leg length of boys, increased hip width of girls, and increased shoulder width of boys helps to explain the increasing performance advantages demonstrated by boys in throwing, jumping, and running activities from 7 years through adulthood.

After adolescence, girls' centers of gravity are lower than those of boys; and for the same height, girls' legs are proportionally shorter (Sinclair, 1973). Again, the implication is that girls would possess more stability and possibly less agility than boys during the adolescent period, giving boys the advantage, for the most part, in physical activity.

Subcutaneous Fat and Body Composition. At all ages girls have more subcutaneous limb and body fat than boys. There is a period of fat loss in the preschool years which is greater for boys, and both sexes gain fat steadily through the elementary school years. In adolescence, both boys and girls continue to increase subcutaneous body fat—girls more than boys. However, while girls steadily increase limb fat, boys decrease it (Tanner, 1962). At all ages boys demonstrate a greater proportion of lean body mass than girls. Boys prove leanest at 16 to 17 years of age, while girls appear most lean at 14 to 15 (Parizkova, 1973).

These differences between the sexes would seem to provide some explanation for why boys perform better than girls in gross motor activities. The leaner the body, the more the body mass can contribute to physical work effort. Leanness, therefore, helps to explain the discrepancies in endurance and physical working capacity seen between the sexes.

Strength. The strength of boys and girls increases similarly as they grow from 6 to 12 years old, although girls score slightly lower in strength than boys (Metheny, 1941; Tuddenham &

Snyder, 1954). After age 12 or 13, however, girls differ markedly from boys. Girls' strength levels and, in some instances, falls off, while boys continue to grow stronger. In fact, for boys, the rate of increase is much greater after the onset of puberty than before. Girls increase most in strength about 2 years earlier than boys, and in some measures, particularly at age 10 to 11, actually outperform boys (Tuddenham & Snyder, 1954).

When body weight is considered, the strength differences between boys and girls grow even more marked after puberty. When corrected for body weight, the postpubescent girl shows virtually no increase in strength. Relative strength, on the other hand, increases dramatically after puberty for boys (Tuddenham & Snyder, 1954).

In short, data regarding strength development in children between 6 and 12 years old do not help account for the discrepancies in their skill performances. Strength data after puberty, however, do help to explain differences in performance.

Physical Working Capacity. Girls do not achieve the capacity for physical work of boys at any age. This sex difference becomes increasingly marked as children grow older. The alkali reserve of males rises at puberty, so that males' blood can absorb greater quantities of lactic acid than can that of females. Females have smaller hearts, less blood volume, lower hemoglobin levels, less available oxygen, and fewer red blood corpuscles than do males. Because of this, particularly after puberty, women generally cannot match men in their capacity to perform work (Adams, Linde, & Hisazumi, 1961a, 1961b; Alderman, 1969; Astrand & Rodahl, 1970; Cumming & Cumming, 1963; DeRiso, 1967; Eichorn, 1970). Superior performance in endurance events is explained to a large extent by these facts of physiology.

Cardiovascular Respiratory Endurance. Maximum oxygen intake tests are generally considered the most valid method of assessing cardiovascular respiratory fitness. Maximum oxygen intake improves with age to 13 years. In fact, when maximal oxygen intake values are corrected for body size, children have scores equal to, or higher than, those of adults. After 13 years, the scores of males increase more rapidly than those of females; from this point boys generally demonstrate significantly better cardiovascular respiratory fitness than do girls. Some studies have even shown girls' performances after age 13 to decrease (Astrand, 1952). Cardiovascular respiratory differences between the sexes provide a partial explanation for males' superior endurance performances.

Flexibility. Studies of 6- through 18-year-old girls show increases in flexibility on most measures to age 12, and decreases in flexibility each year thereafter (Hupprich & Sigerseth, 1950). Though no studies exist, it is likely that flexibility performances for boys are similar. Although research within sex groups indicates that length of body parts does not affect flexibility scores, it is generally accepted that girls have greater potential for flexibility after puberty on such measures as trunk flexion because of their lower center of gravity and shorter leg length.

Sex-Role Expectations

Although structural and physiological differences between the sexes provide powerful explanations for many of the discrepancies in the gross motor performances of males and females (particularly during and following adolescence), they are not, in themselves, sufficient explanations for the consistent differences seen in childhood. Socialization processes are apparently responsible for many of the performance differences between young boys and girls.

Our society's cultural patterns celebrate strength and endurance—both characteristics predominantly associated with males. We characterize our females, for the most part, as dependent, passive, fragile, nonaggressive, noncompetitive, accepting, supportive, and emotionally pliable beings; while our men are depicted as independent, agressive, strong, enduring, courageous, active, disciplined, and emotionally controlled. Women in our society are to some extent programmed not to try, and have almost been conditioned to fear success. In our society, a girl is expected to maintain a "feminine image" in her dress, tone of voice, gesticulations, and general movement behavior.

The socialization process which inculcates these values begins in the first year of life. Goldberg and Lewis (1969) illustrated these early effects in their study of the behavior of 13-month-old boys and girls in interaction with their mothers. They found that girls were more dependent than boys, showed less exploratory behavior, and played more quietly. Boys played with toys that required more gross motor activity. They tended to be more vigorous and to run more in their play. Girls proved more reluctant than boys to leave their mothers, staying near them during play and seeking physical reassurance more often.

In early childhood, parents are predominantly responsible for socializing their children. Parental behavior acquires reinforcement value which allows it to influence and regulate children's behavior. Both parents are likely to reinforce those behaviors they consider sex-role appropriate, and the child learns what are appropriate sex-role behaviors independent of any internal motive—just as he or she learns any appropriate response rewarded by parents. Fling and Manosevitz (1972) have demonstrated that parents discourage cross-sexed play interests in boys more than in girls and that parents of the same sex as their child encourage sex-typing more than do opposite-sexed parents. As the child becomes older, the rules for this class of reinforced behaviors become clear and the child develops internal guides which cause him or her not only to continue behaviors earlier reinforced by parents, but even to incorporate new behavior patterns into the scheme which are consistent with past parental expectations and in keeping with the behavior expectations of other newly significant people (Kagan, 1964, Mischel, 1966; Roberts & Sutton-Smith, 1962; Spencer, 1970).

We know that children learn their sex roles very early and that assignment of these roles just after birth is continually reinforced as children grow older. We know that these learnings and reinforcements do influence human behavior. Yet when we examine research literature to define the relationship that certainly must exist between movement behavior and sex-role expectations, we find little is known. What information is available falls into three general areas: (1) game preferences of young children, (2) children's perceptions of the appropriateness of motor activities for each of the sexes, and (3) the influence of sex-labeling of games on children's game performances and game preferences.

Game Preferences of Children

The game preferences of children provide insight into the relationship between sex-role expectations and movement behavior. To some extent, they reflect the learning of appropriate sex-role behaviors.

Sutton-Smith and Rosenberg (1961) studied data regarding game preferences that had been collected (a) in 1896 in Worcester, Mass., on 1929 children who were between the ages of 6 and 18, (b) in 1898 in South Carolina on 8718 children who were between 6 and 18, (c) in 1921 in the Bay Area of California on 474 children between 6 and 17, and (d) in 1959 in northwest Ohio on 2689 children between 9 and 15. Diverse games were included in the various studies (e.g., baseball, football, hide-and-seek, tag, marbles, cards, drop-the-handkerchief, Simon says, fox and geese, jacks, jump rope, hopscotch). Among their findings, Sutton-Smith and Rosenberg noted that over the decades the game preferences of girls have become increasingly like those of boys (a finding not unexpected in light of the changes in women's roles in American culture during the last 80 years), and that boys' game preferences have become increasingly circumscribed. Boys appear to be steadily lowering their preferences for games that have anything to do with girls' play. They seem to have reduced the range of games of individual and team skill and the organized sports to which they will devote their time. This limiting condition tends to contribute to clear-cut definitions of appropriate boys' behavior. However, it penalizes the boys who are better suited to other activities.

Sutton-Smith, Rosenberg, and Morgan (1963) administered a play inventory of 180 items to 1900 children in grades 3 through 6 which contained items identified in previous research as either masculine or feminine. They found that girls showed an increasing interest in masculine items through all these grades—with the major changes occurring between grades 3 and 4. Girls' preferences for masculine items apparently increase with increasing age, and there is no tendency in the upper elementary grades to reverse this trend.

Children's Perceptions of the Appropriateness of Motor Activities for Each Sex

Children's perceptions of activities as being most appropriate either for boys or girls also provide some insight into the relationship between sex-role expectations and the movement behavior of children. They, too, reflect the learning of appropriate sex-role behavior.

Herkowitz (1976) asked 360 children equally divided as to age and sex among preschool, second grade, fifth grade, eighth grade, eleventh grade, and university sophomores, to view each of 35 slides depicting motor activities being performed by a stick figure having no distinguishing sex characteristics. After each figure was presented, children were asked to indicate whether they felt each activity was a boys' activity, a girls' activity, or a boys' or girls' activity by marking one of the three sections on an answer sheet depicting the same stick figure representations, but with sex-distinguishing features.

Among the statistically significant findings: (1) there was a tendency to perceive motor activities as more appropriate for both sexes than as appropriate only for one sex or the other; (2) the tendency to type motor activities as appropriate for both boys and girls was stronger in females than in males; (3) activities were ordered according to the degree to which they were sex-typed, with the most strongly sex-typed activities perceived as boys' activities by the majority of students; (4) disagreements between the sexes as to how activities should be typed occurred less frequently with increasing age; (5) differences among age/grade only in typing existed, but appeared to be more a result of preschoolers' tendencies to select the *girls' activity* and *boys' activity* categories rather than the *boys' or girls' activity* category more than did older children participating in the study. The preschoolers did not seem able to deal effectively with the three-category data.

Influence of Sex-Typed Labels on Children's Performances and Preferences

Surprisingly little research has been done on the direct influence of sex-appropriate or sex-inappropriate labeling of activities on children's subsequent motor behavior and preferences. Liebert, McCall, and Hanratty (1971) experimentally manipulated the sex-typed information of two groups of toys. First grade children were told that a group of toys were preferred by their own sex and that a second group were preferred by the opposite sex. The children were then asked to choose the toys which they preferred. Data revealed that when children were told which toys their own sex preferred, they matched preferences. Their preferences were not influenced, however, by knowledge of what the opposite sex preferred. In short, the data indicated that same-sex labels were more effective in influencing toy preference than opposite-sex labels.

Stein, Pohly, and Mueller (1971) examined achievement in sixth grade children as a function of sex label of the task. Children were presented with three paper-and-pencil tasks involving words and pictures. The tasks were labeled masculine, feminine, and neutral, and each task received each label. Each child was given a total of 10 minutes to work on all three tasks. Results indicated that boys spent most of the time working on the male task, an intermediate amount of time on the neutral task, and the least time on the female task. Girls, however, spent about the same amount of time on each task.

Montemayor (1974) examined 6- through 8-year-old children's performances in and attraction to a game as a function of sex-typed labels. The child played a game called *Mr. Munchie,* which was labeled either sex-appropriately, sex-neutrally, or sex-inappropriately. Munchie was a clown's head with a spiral-shaped rod, 12 inches long, with a clown hat attached to the top. The game was played by pulling the clown's head up the rod to his hat. When his head was released, it moved down the rod until it was attached to the body again. All this took approximately 13 seconds. The child was to throw as many plastic marbles as possible into Mr. Munchie's body before the head had descended. A six-point scale was used to measure the attractiveness of the game. Numbers of marbles gotten in were the performance scores assessed. For both boys and girls, performance was best when the game was labeled sex-appropriate, intermediate when no sex label was given, and lowest when it was labeled as sex-inappropriate. For attractiveness, the appropriate- and neutral-label conditions were similar, and both were higher than in the inappropriate condition. The effect of labeling on performance was equal among both boys and girls. Scores for boys and girls were about the mirror image of each other.

In comparing the studies, it would seem that when asked to choose between male and female objects, girls choose both male and female objects equally, while boys choose male objects and reflect female objects—at least on the sixth grade level. Among first graders, same-sex preference labels seem to influence performance more than opposite-sex preference labels. When asked to perform in an activity which is clearly labeled sex-appropriate or sex-inappropriate, both boys and girls perform as they believe to be consistent with their own sex. Future researchers may want to consider choice of task, task performance, and task preference as separate indices of sex-role influences.

Findings

The fairly consistent motor performance advantage of boys can only partially be explained by structural and physiological sex differences. Socialization seems to offer a more potent explanation for performance discrepancies between the sexes. Investigations regarding children's game preferences, their perceptions of sex-appropriate motor behavior, and the influence of sex labels on motor performance and motor activity attractiveness clearly demonstrate the effect of socialization on performance. on performance.

What now seem appropriate questions for educators and researchers to ponder are:

1. To what degree does sex-labeling by same-sex or opposite-sex parents influence motor performance and preference early in life?
2. To what degree does sex-labeling by same-sex or opposite-sex peers influence motor performance and preference at different ages?
3. To what degree and how do physical education teachers sex-label activities, and how much does their labeling influence the motor performances and preferences of their students?
4. Does sex-typing behavior change with social class?
5. What are the nature and dynamics of the sanctions imposed on children for inappropriate sex-role behavior in motor activity?
6. Should one sex-label activity to help children through the process of gender identification, or should one not sex-label in any way (Mischel, 1970; Werner, 1972)?

REFERENCES

American Association for Health, Physical Education, and Recreation. *Youth Fitness Test Manual.* Washington, D. C.: American Association for Health, Physical Education, and Recreation, 1965.

Adams, F. H., Linde, L. M., & Hisazumi, M. The physical working capacity of normal school children, I. *Pediatrics,* 1961 (*a*), *28,* 55.

Adams, F. H., Linde, L. M., & Hisazumi, M. The physical working capacity of normal school children, II. *Pediatrics,* 1961 (*b*), *28,* 243.

Alderman, R. B. Age and sex differences in PWC 170 of Canadian school children. *Research Quarterly,* 1969, *40,* 1-5.

Astrand, P. O. *Experimental Studies of Working Capacity in Relation to Sex and Age.* Copenhagen: Mucksgoaard, 1952.

Astrand, P. O., & Rodahl, K. *Textbook of Work Physiology.* New York: McGraw-Hill, 1970.

Cumming, G. R., & Cumming, P. M. Working capacity of normal children tested on a bicycle ergometer. *Canadian Medical Association Journal,* 1963, *88,* 51-55.

DeRiso, J. D. Assessing the PWC of elementary school children. Unpublished master's thesis, University of Pittsburgh, 1967.

Eichorn, D. Physiological development. In Mussen, P.H., ed. *Carmichael's Manual of Child Psychology,* vol. I. New York: Wiley, 1970.

Espenschade, A. Motor development. In Johnson, W. R., ed. *Science and Medicine of Exercise and Sports.* New York: Harper & Row, 1960.

Fling, S., & Manosevitz, M. Sex typing in nursery school children's play interests. *Developmental Psychology,* 1972, *7,* 146-152.

Glassow, R. B., & Kruse, P. Motor performances of girls. *Research Quarterly,* 1960, *31,* 426-433.

Goldberg, S., & Lewis, M. Play behavior in the year-old infant: Early sex differences. *Child Development,* 1969, *40,* 21-31.

Halverson, L. E., & Roberton, M. A. A study of motor pattern development in young children. Paper presented at the research section meeting of the American Association for Health, Physical Education, and Recreation National Convention, Chicago, Ill., March, 1966.

Hanson, M. Motor performance testing of elementary school age children. Unpublished doctoral dissertation, University of Washington, 1965.

Herkowitz, J. Sex-appropriateness of motor activities. Paper presented at the research section meeting of the American Association for Health, Physical Education, and Recreation National Convention, Milwaukee, Wis., April, 1976.

Hoadley, D. A study of the catching ability of children in grades one to four. Unpublished master's thesis, University of Iowa, 1941.

Hupprich, F. L., & Sigerseth, P. O. Specificity of flexibility in girls. *Research Quarterly,* 1950, *21,* 25-33.

Jenkins, L. A comparative study of motor achievements of children of five, six and seven years of age. *Contributions to Education,* Teachers College, Columbia University, No. 414, 1930.

Johnson, R. Measurements of achievement in fundamental skills of elementary school children. *Research Quarterly,* 1962, *33,* 94-104.

Jones, F. A descriptive and mechanical analysis of throwing skills of children. Unpublished master's thesis, University of Wisconsin, 1951.

Kagan, J. Acquisition and significance of sex-typing and sex-role identity. In Hoffman, M., & Hoffman, L. eds. *Review of Child Development Research.* New York: Russell Sage Foundation, 1964.

Keogh, J. Motor performance of elementary school children. Unpublished manuscript, University of California at Los Angeles, 1965.

Latchaw, M. Measuring selected motor skills in fourth, fifth, and sixth grades. *Research Quarterly,* 1954, *25,* 439-449.

Liebert, R. M., McCall, R. B., & Hanratty, M. A. Effects of sex-typed information on children's toy preferences. *Journal of Genetic Psychology,* 1971, *119,* 133-136.

Metheny, E. Breathing capacity and grip strength of preschool children. *University of Iowa Studies in Child Welfare,* 1941, *18,* 1.

Mischel, W. A social learning view of sex differences in behavior. In Maccoby, E., ed. *The Development of Sex Differences.* Stanford, Cal.: Stanford University Press, 1966.

Mischel, W. Sex-typing and socialization. In Mussen, P. H., ed. *Carmichael's Manual of Child Psychology.* New York: Wiley, 1970.

Montemayor, R. Children's performance in a game and their attraction to it as a function of sex-typed labels. *Child Development,* 1974, *45,* 152-156.

Parizkova, J. Body composition and exercise. In Rarick, L. R., ed. *Physical Activity.* New York: Academic Press, 1973.

Roberts, J., & Sutton-Smith, B. Child training and game involvement. *Ethnology,* 1962, *1,* 164-185.

Rosenberg. B., & Sutton-Smith, B. A revised conception of masculine-feminine differences in play activities. *Journal of Genetic Psychology,* 1960, *96.* 165-170.

Seils, L. The relationship between measures of physical growth and gross motor performance of primary-grade children. *Research Quarterly,* 1951, *22,* 244-260.

Sinclair, D. *Human Growth After Birth.* London: Oxford University Press, 1973.

Spencer, T. Sex role learning in early childhood. In Hartup, W., ed. *The Young Child: Reviews of Research.* Washington, D.C.: National Association for the Education of Children, 1970.

Stein, A., Pohly, S., & Mueller, E. The influence of masculine, feminine, and neutral tasks on children's achievement behavior, expectancies of success, and attainment values. *Child Development,* 1971, *42,* 195-207.

Sutton-Smith, B., & Rosenberg, G. Sixty years of historical change in the game preferences of American children. *Journal of American Folklore,* 1961, *74,* 17-46.

Sutton-Smith. B., Rosenberg, B. G., & Morgan, Jr., E. Development of sex differences in play choices during preadolescence. *Child Development,* 1963, *34,* 119-126.

Tanner, J. M. *Growth at Adolescence.* London: Blackwell Scientific Publications. Ltd., 1962.

Tanner, J. M., Whitehouse, R. H., & Takaishi, M. Standards from birth to maturity for height, weight, height velocity, and weight velocity, British children, 1965. *Archives of Disease in Childhood,* 1966, *41,* 454-471, 613-635.

Tuddenham, R. D., & Snyder, M. M. *Physical Growth of California Boys and Girls from Birth to Eighteen Years.* Los Angeles: University of California Press, 1954.

Walker, R. Measuring masculinity and femininity by children's game choices. *Child Development,* 1964, *35,* 961-971.

Werner, P. The role of the physical educator in gender identification. *Physical Educator,* 1972, *29,* 27-28.

Wild, M. The behavior pattern of throwing and some observations concerning its course of development in children. *Research Quarterly,* 1938. *9,* 20-24.

6

Memory Processes in the Early Acquisition of Motor Skills

JANE E. CLARK

Research in motor development has focused primarily on the determination of universal sequences of fundamental or phylogenetic movement patterns. Early research identified pattern-specific milestones and chronologies for movement behaviors such as locomotion (Shirley, 1931; McGraw, 1940), prehension (Halverson, 1931), swimming (McGraw, 1939), and overhand throwing (Wild, 1937). It was assumed implicitly, if not explicitly, that a person's movement patterns "unfolded" or matured and that those behaviors were universal to all men. Developmental questions were directed not toward *why* or *how* the phenomena occurred, but rather toward *what* was occurring (that is, the content of the sequence). As a result, we have little process-oriented research on the development of motor behavior. Although studies on the motor skills of adults abound, few researchers have concentrated on the age-related processes or mechanisms of motor skill performance and acquisition.

Assumption of an Information Processing Model

While we recognize that the descriptive and normative approach to understanding the development of motor control was necessary, it is argued here that present inquiries should concentrate on clarifying what underlying processes are changing as the child gains control of his movement. One possible approach to refocusing developmental questions is an information processing model of man. Such a conceptualization would not only provide us with a substantial data bank of information (drawn from the voluminous research on adults), but more importantly would permit us to examine the underlying processes ultimately responsible for the changing movement behavior we observe. In fact, the suggestion of using such a theoretical framework in motor development is not new; Williams (1973) and Connolly (1970) have both proposed its adoption.

It is our goal here to examine one aspect or component of information processing, the *memory process*. Such a review and analysis can help to provide information on a process which may be changing throughout life and consequently may be affecting motor performance and motor skill acquisition. Although much of the research presented here has not been conducted on motor memory, it should nevertheless suggest possible implications and directions for future research questions concerning the recall and reproduction of motor responses in children.

Our focus in this chapter has been limited to *early development* of memory processes, rather than a comprehensive life-span perspective. Thus, the chapter examines the development of memory in the child, emphasizing how this process may affect the development of motor behavior.

Memory

All conceptualizations of man or child as an information processing system include *memory*. This mechanism provides man with the capacity to maintain information after the stimuli or information is no longer present. Although there are many theories of memory processing, most view memory not a a unitary process but rather as a three-stage system involving several processes. Generally, the three stages or stores are *short-term sensory store* (STSS), *short-term memory* (STM), and *long-term memory* (LTM). Several processes are postulated for maintaining information in and extracting information from the various stores; they are: *encoding, rehearsal,* and *retrieval.*

The short-term sensory store maintains all environmental stimuli for a very short time (approximately ½ second after the physical signal has disappeared). It allows the system to operate and extract information from the stimuli changing and disappearing within that specific modality. One's short-term memory retains a limited amount of information on immediate experiences for approximately half a minute. Information in short-term memory has been interpreted and encoded from the short-term sensory store and will require rehearsal to be maintained. Probably the most important memory store, however, is long-term memory. It is this capacity which permits us to keep and later retrieve information gained minutes, days, or even years ago.

Developmentally, the importance of memory seems obvious. If there are age-related changes in this mechanism, it would constitute one possibility for explaining age differences in motor performance. But where might these changes occur? Does the young child have limitations in the capacity of any or all the various memory stores? Or is the change occurring within processes of encoding, rehearsal, or retrieval of information? Or simply, is the young child's limitation one of an inadequate long-term memory, his not having had as many antecedent experiences as his adult counterpart?

Short-Term Sensory Store

In the adult, STSS has been demonstrated for visual stimuli (Averbach and Coriell, 1961; Sperling, 1960). After a brief exposure of many visual stimuli, subjects are usually able to report only a few of the items. The brief visual representation fades quickly, limiting the subject's recall to only a few items in the complete report paradigm. However, by using a partial report method, it can be demonstrated that subjects actually have all stimuli available up to ½ second after the signal has disappeared.

Using the partial report method with 5-, 8-, 11-, and 21-year-olds, Sheingold (1973) was able to demonstrate that there were no age differences in the initial intake of visual stimuli. The young child's short-term sensory store for visual stimuli was not different from that of older subjects. However, age differences in recall did occur when the interval between stimulus offset and recall was delayed. Older subjects appeared to employ an active strategy for encoding the items which younger subjects were not using.

Apparently the young child (of at least 5 years) receives as much visual information into the system initially as does the older subject. However, if he must maintain this information for a longer period of time, his recall declines more quickly than that of his older counterpart. This age difference is not in STSS, but in short-term memory.

Short-Term Memory

As noted earlier, for the system to maintain information over a lengthened interval, information in STSS must be transformed or encoded into the short-term memory (STM), which has an approximate 30-second capacity. It is at this point in the memory systems that age differences begin to appear. For example, in an earlier study by Sheingold and her colleagues (Haith, Morrison, Sheingold, & Mindes, 1970), 5-year-olds and adults were shown two, three, or four familiar geometric forms for 150 msec. Upon recall, the 5-year-olds were able to remember less than two items out of those presented, whereas adults routinely could recall all forms even in the four-item presentation.

If there is no initial age-related difference in the amount of visual information that enters the system, why, after a delay before recall, do age differences appear? Several possibilities exist. First, there may be differences in the encoding process. For a person to retain information for longer than a ½ second, he or she must transfer information from STSS to STM. For example, if the initial stimuli are visual, subsequent encoding may transform the information into verbal code.

Haith (1971) and others have suggested that the young child may be using a different encoding strategy than older subjects. Instead of using the verbal code employed by older subjects, the young subject may be employing a visual code which may have less capacity or be less easily rehearsed, both of which would affect his or her performance. Many studies have demonstrated that younger children do not employ verbal labels or verbal rehearsal in memory tasks (Flavell, Beach, & Chinsky, 1966; Keeney, Cannizzo, & Flavell, 1967; Hagen & Kingsley, 1968; and Conrad, 1971). If prompted to use overt verbalizations, their performance does improve; however, they do not maintain such a strategy without prompting (Keeney, Cannizzo, & Flavell, 1967; Kingsley and Hagen, 1969; Hagen, Hargrave, & Ross, 1973). The evidence would support, therefore, possible age differences in the encoding of visual material. It also suggests differences in *rehearsal,* which has been shown to be an important process in getting information into long-term memory.

A second variable which may affect children's performance on STM tasks is *attention.* Sroufe (Sroufe, 1971; Sroufe, Sonies, West, & Wright, 1973) has physiological evidence on cardiac deceleration within a fixed foreperiod prior to stimulus onset which suggests that young children do not reliably maintain a stable attentive state of responding. There may well be a developmental change in the ability to maintain attention. If, as some argue, attentional processes contribute to those items which enter the STM store, then developmental differences in attention could account, in part, for memory differences in the young children.

And finally, another variable related to attention which may affect STM is the scanning of the visual array presented to the children. It has been found that younger children do not disregard the irrelevant and uninformative stimuli present in an array as do the older subjects (Druker & Hagen, 1969; Hagen, 1967). Further, the younger subjects do not seem to scan the array for those items or features which may be most useful to them in successfully completing their task (Vurpillot, 1968).

Clearly, age differences do exist in STM for visually-presented stimuli. Such differences suggest that possibly there are age-related functions or changes occurring in the way information is encoded and rehearsed, and these changes have a twofold effect on motor skill acquisition. First, visual stimuli are an important source of information to most motor skill performance, and differences in what is remembered in the visual array will certainly affect this performance. For example, after hitting a ball, the child must remember where the ball went—how far and in which direction—in order to use this information to either repeat or modify subsequent hits. Second, if there are developmental changes in encoding processes for visual information, is it possible that such changes may occur in the encoding and rehearsal processes for movement information? The latter implication is of particular interest, for one of the more intriguing questions for research on early skill acquisition raised by the examination of memory processes is *how movement is remembered.* Particularly, are there developmental differences in such processes?

Short-Term Motor Memory

Unfortunately, we have no studies which have directly addressed short-term motor memory (STMM) developmentally. There are a few experiments, however, which may lend some insight into the process of remembering movements. Zaichkowsky (1974), in examining the development of perceptual motor sequencing abilities, pursued the possibility that STM may be a limiting factor in its development. Using a task similar to tasks of serial recall of verbal material, Zaichkowsky presented 5-, 7-, and 9-year-olds with a sequence of lights paired with responding pedals which were flashed on in either a random or organized sequence. Following the last light flash, subjects were to reproduce the sequence by hitting the corresponding pedals in the appropriate order. In the organized pattern where lights were presented in a clockwise sequence (i. e., left hand, right hand, right foot, left foot, etc., LH, RH, RF, LF), all subjects including the youngest made fewer errors than in the random pattern condition (LH, RF, LF, RF, RH, LF, LH, RH). Under both pattern conditions, however, there were age differences; 5-year-olds made more errors than the other two older groups. An age x pattern organization interaction indicated that the age differences were magnified by the random pattern condition. In the random or nonsense pattern sequence, Zaichkowsky suggests older subjects may have been covertly verbalizing or rehearsing the order, a strategy which the 5-year-olds did not employ.

One criticism of the Zaichkowsky study which requires further discussion is whether or not this task represented a STM phenomenon. There is evidence on serial recall tasks which indicates that items early in the list are remembered because they pass from STM to LTM through rehearsal (Murdock, 1962; Waugh & Norman, 1965; Ellis, 1969). Since the task was to recall the sequence in order, items at the end of the list, which usually represents those items in STM, were lost probably due to interference. When ordered recall is not required, subjects usually remember items late in the list by immediately retrieving them from STM (referred to as "recency") and those early in the list, which are retrieved from LTM (referred to as "primacy"). By insisting on an ordered recall, Zaichkowsky found primacy but not recency. Further, the memorization in this task had a strong verbal component. As has been pointed out earlier, older subjects employ verbal encoding and rehearsal that younger subjects do not use, and these strategies may aid the older subjects' recall performance on items early in the sequence. To examine possible encoding differences for movements, this strong verbal component should be reduced to a minimum. Nonetheless, Zaichkowsky's data do suggest age differences in motor tasks requiring sequential order.

In a study employing a task closely resembling short-term motor memory tasks used with adults, Smothergill (1973) investigated spatial localization across ages. He found no age differences for localizing (i. e., pointing at) targets present in the visual field. If, however, the target was presented and then removed, age differences increased with delays in the interval prior to recall. The older subjects (in this study 9- and 10-year-olds, and adults) were superior to the younger children (6- and 7-year-olds) in remembering the target's position. No differential effects were found for accuracy of recall and the mode of target presentation (either proprioceptively, visually, or proprioceptively and visually). However, visual and visual-proprioceptive presentation were recalled more accurately than proprioceptive-alone presentations in all groups.

Two other studies, one by Rieber (1968) and the other by Whiting and Cockerill (1972), offer further evidence of possible age-related differences in short-term motor memory. Although neither was designed specifically to answer questions concerning developmental changes in STMM, they do provide some data on children's recall of a force-producing movement. Rieber employed a pin-ball type machine in which his subjects (5-, 7-, and 9-year-olds) had to get a ball into the hole at the end of the runway. The apparatus had a plunger with a pointer and scale constructed so that the subject could have precise information concerning the appropriate force to be applied by the plunger. Subjects were either permitted to see this scale or were not. Overall, the two youngest groups' performance differed from the older group's. Also, having the indicator and seeing their own hand on the plunger improved performance over performance without such cues. Of interest to STMM is the "blind" performance of all the groups when they could not see the scale and indicator, relying on proprioceptive feedback and knowledge of results, that is, feedback from moving and seeing where the ball went. Rieber reports only 10 percent of the kindergarten and second-grade groups learned the "blind" task while approximately 25 to 40 percent of the older group learned it.

In the other study (Whiting and Cockerill, 1972) the youngest subjects (5-year-olds) were unable accurately to project a toy car up an incline to a specified spot which they saw prior to, but not at, the moment the toy was released. Older subjects were able to perform the task.

We have little systematic research on STMM in children today. We do have, however, some clues and questions that might provide a basis for future research. For example, Smothergill's study suggests that when recall is delayed, young children do not remember end locations of movement as well as older subjects. Even under conditions of seeing and being guided to the criterion target, younger subjects simply do not recall movements accurately after delayed retention intervals. STMM research on adults has suggested that end location is an important cue in the recall of movements and does not deteriorate in an unfilled retention interval (Laabs, 1973; Russell, 1974). What might be the cause of possible age-related differences of spatial localization?

Smothergill suggested that the younger children's poorer performance may have been *not* the result of a STM deficit, but the loss of an "attentive readiness" state. However, one might also argue that in a long unfilled retention interval, older subjects rehearsed the encoded location and the younger subjects did not. The older children may have attached verbal labels to the presented location (such as "just right of center") or, as Williams (1973) has suggested, they may be positing the target into a well-established "frame of reference"—a reference system which the young child has not fully developed yet. Clearly, more systematic research is necessary to separate out the variables which may affect the accuracy of movement reproduction.

What then, is the importance of short-term memory to early skill acquisition? The studies presented indicate that there are developmental differences in STM, and the implication of these differences should be clear. An accurate short-term store is a necessary component of an information processing system. Experiences or movements in the immediate past are necessary for immediate corrections or adjustments. In throwing a ball at a target, for example, a miss might be made to the right. On the next attempt, the subject adjusts to the left. If you cannot remember the consequences of the previous movement, however, you are likely to continue to make the same error. Without memory, you are not likely to improve no matter how much you practice.

Long-Term Memory

Although we have questioned how one remembers one's previous movement, we might also ask how one remembers movements such as swimming or bicycling which may remain unpracticed or unhearsed for months or years. How do such patterns get into LTM? How are they encoded or represented? Very little research has been conducted on LTM—despite its obvious importance.

Rehearsal is one way in which movements get into long-term memory. Zaichkowsky's data suggest that the young child can get movements early in a sequence into LTM, although they make more errors than older children. Overt practice, repeating a specific movement over and over again, provides a motor rehearsal young children display every day. In fact, motor skills are probably the most overpracticed or overlearned skills of man.

But although we know we rehearse movements often, we still do not know how they are encoded or represented in LTM. It does not seem difficult to think what you might do if given a bicycle and told to ride it; you would just get on and off you would go. But how did you retrieve the motor commands for such a response? One possible model presently being given new consideration is a conceptualization of Bartlett's (1932) which he labeled *schema* (see Evans, 1967; Schmidt, 1975). Essentially, within this model *rules* for movement generation are stored —not the specific patterns or memory traces. This "schema" model would suggest that movement experiences be varied to induce the elaboration of generative rules. When a movement is required, these stored rules are retrieved to produce the neccessary movement.

Another conceptualization which Bruner (1973) eludes to and Pew (1970) specifies, is *goal-oriented memory*. This type of notion could be incorporated with "schema" in the sense that retrieval or storage labels were based on the *purpose* of the required movement, not on a verbal label for the movement. The process would then consist of specifying the goal, and the rules for the movement response appropriate to the goal would be retrieved.

Obviously, we need more research on long-term memory. Without it, we will not be able to understand the age-related changes in motor skill acquisition. In particular, are differences in performance among age groups a function of an experience deficit (that is, a quantitative difference) or of a qualitative difference in LTM processing? A schema theory would posit that children have fewer generative rules because they have not had as many varied experiences as older subjects, but such a postulation requires further experimentation.

Summary

In summary, there appears to be evidence of age-related differences in the three stages of memory and their processes. Clearly, memory plays a key role in the acquisition and performance of motor skills. Information regarding developmental differences in memory, therefore, suggests at least a possible process responsible for the differences observed in the motor behavior of children and adults. To understand more about the development of motor control, researchers must continue to pursue a process-oriented approach to motor development.

REFERENCES

Averbach, E., & Coriell, A. S. Short-term memory in vision. *Bell System Technical Journal*, 1961, *40*, 309-328.

Bartlett, F. C. *Remembering*. Cambridge, Eng.: Cambridge University Press, 1932.

Bruner, J. S. Organization of early skilled action. *Child Development*, 1973, *44*, 1-11.

Connolly, K., ed. *Mechanisms of Motor Skill Development*. New York: Academic Press, 1970.

Conrad, R. The chronology of the development of covert speech in children. *Developmental Psychology*, 1971, *5*, 398-405.

Druker, J. F., & Hagen, J. W. Developmental trends in the processing of task-relevant and task-irrelevant information. *Child Development*, 1969, *40*, 371-382.

Ellis, N. R. Evidence for two storage processes in short-term memory. *Journal of Experimental Psychology*, 1969, *80*, 390-391.

Evans, S. H. A brief statement of schema theory. *Psychonomic Science*, 1967, *8*, 87-88.

Flavell, J. H., Beach, D. H., & Chinsky, J. M. Spontaneous verbal rehearsal in a memory task as a function of age. *Child Development*, 1966, *37*, 283-299.

Hagen, J. W. The effect of distraction on selective attention. *Child Development*, 1967, *38*, 685-694.

Hagen, J. W., Hargrave, S., & Ross, W. Prompting and rehearsal in short-term memory. *Child Development*, 1973, *44*, 201-204.

Hagen, J W., & Kingsley, P. Labeling effects in short-term memory. *Child Development*, 1968, *39*, 113-121.

Haith, M. M. Developmental changes in visual information processing and short-term visual memory. *Human Development*, 1971, *14*, 249-261.

Haith, M. M., Morrison, F. J., Sheingold, K., & Mindes, P. Short-term memory for visual information in children and adults. *Journal of Experimental Child Psychology*, 1970, *9*, 454-469.

Halverson, H. M. An experimental study of prehension in infants by means of systematic cinema records. *Genetic Psychology Monographs*, 1931, *10*, 107-286.

Keeney, T. J., Cannizzo, S. R., & Flavell, J. J. Spontaneous and induced verbal rehearsal in a recall task. *Child Development*, 1967, *38*, 953-966.

Kingsley, P., & Hagen, J. Induced versus spontaneous rehearsal in short-term memory in nursery school children. *Developmental Psychology*, 1969, *1*, 40-46.

Laabs, G. J. Retention characteristics of different reproduction cues in motor short-term memory. *Journal of Experimental Psychology,* 1973. *100,* 168-177.

McGraw, M. B. Neuromuscular development of the human infant as exemplified in the achievement of erect locomotion. *Journal of Pediatrics,* 1940, *17,* 747-771.

McGraw, M. B. Swimming behavior of the human infant. *Journal of Pediatrics,* 1939, *15,* 485-490.

Murdock, B. B., Jr. The serial effect of free recall. *Journal of Experimental Psychology,* 1962, *64,* 482-488.

Pew, R. W. Toward a process-oriented theory of human skilled performance. *Journal of Motor Behavior,* 1970, *2,* 8-24.

Reese, H. W. Models of memory and models of development. *Human Development,* 1973, *16,* 397-416.

Rieber, M. Mediational aids and motor skill learning in children. *Child Development,* 1968, *39,* 559-567.

Russell, D. G. Location cues and the generation of movement. Paper presented to the North American Society for the Psychology of Sport and Physical Activity, Anaheim, Cal., 1974.

Schmidt, R. A. A schema theory of discrete motor skill learning. *Psychological Review,* 1975, *82,* 225-260.

Sheingold, K. Developmental differences in intake and storage of visual information. *Journal of Experimental Child Psychology,* 1973, *16,* 1-11.

Shiffrin, R. M., & Atkinson, R. C. Storage and retrieval processes in long-term memory. *Psychological Review,* 1969, *76,* 179-193.

Shirley, M. *First Two Years: A Study of Twenty-Five Babies.* Vol. I. Minneapolis: University of Minnesota Press, 1931.

Smothergill, D. W. Accuracy and variability in localization of spatial targets at three age levels. *Developmental Psychology,* 1973, *8,* 62-66.

Sperling, G. The information available in brief visual presentations. *Psychological Monographs,* 1960, *74* (whole no. 11).

Sroufe, L. A. Age changes in cardiac deceleration within a fixed foreperiod reaction-time task: an index of attention. *Developmental Psychology,* 1971, *5,* 338-343.

Sroufe, L. A., Sonies, B. C., West, W. D., & Wright, F. S. Anticipatory heart rate deceleration and reaction time in children with and without referral for learning disability. *Child Development,* 1973, *44,* 267-273.

Vurpillot, E. The development of scanning strategies and their relation to visual differentiation. *Journal of Experimental Child Psychology*, 1968, *6*, 632-650.

Waugh, N. C., & Norman, D. A. Primary memory. *Psychological Review*, 1965, *72*, 89-104.

Whiting, H. T. A., & Cockerill, I. M. The development of a simple ballistic skill with and without visual control. *Journal of Motor Behavior*, 1972, *4*, 155-162.

Wild, M. R. The behavior pattern of throwing and some observations concerning its course of development in children. Unpublished doctoral dissertation, University of Wisconsin, Madison, 1937.

Williams, H. G. Perceptual-motor development as a function of information processing. In Wade, M. G., & Martens, R., eds. *Psychology of Motor Behavior and Sport*, Proceedings of the North American Society for Psychology of Sport and Physical Activity, 1973.

Zaichkowsky, L. D. The development of perceptual motor sequencing ability. *Journal of Motor Behavior*, 1974, *6*, 255-261.

Part III

**Applications:
Environments, Curricula
and Evaluation**

7

The Design and Evaluation of Playspaces for Children

JACQUELINE HERKOWITZ

Preschool and primary school children are in the midst of a growth and development period characterized by significant changes. Alterations in body proportions, stature, weight, bone ossification, muscle and fat distribution, heart rate, physical working capacity, cardiovascular-respiratory fitness, strength, flexibility, figure-ground perception, size constancy, body image, depth perception, conceptions about space and time, conceptions about significant others, interests, activity preferences, and motor skills all work to make this a period of plasticity in which children are enormously susceptible to their environment. Yet this plasticity is a two-edged sword; while a youngster is highly responsive to the challenge of an appropriate environment, he is equally susceptible to the deprivations of an impoverished one.

Indoor and outdoor playspaces can be a significant part of a child's environment, and their design should not be taken lightly. Unfortunately, little useful theory or research is available to provide guidelines (Ellis, 1970; Wuellner, 1970). Consequently, playspace design has, for the most part, been a function of hunch, intuition, unsystematic observation, and what is available in equipment catalogs.

The purpose of this paper is to share a theoretically based rationale for the design of playspaces, examine a variety of environmental elements influencing the behavior of children in light of that rationale, and, finally, to suggest techniques that may be useful in evaluating playspaces. When appropriate and available, research will be cited.

Theoretical Conceptions of Play

Four recent theories of play seem particularly capable of providing direction for those interested in designing playspaces (Ellis, 1971). *Developmentalism* is the first theory. It conceives of play as caused by the way in which a child's mind and body develop. Play occurs when the child can impose on reality his own conceptions and constraints. This explanation assumes that play involves the body and intellect, that as a result of play the body and intellect increase in complexity, that this process in the human being can be separated into stages, and that children pass through these stages in order.

Learning is the second theory. It conceives of play as being caused by the normal processes that produce learning. This theory assumes that the child acts to increase the probability of pleasant events and to decrease the probability of unpleasant events, that the environment is a complex of pleasant and unpleasant effects, and that the environment selects and energizes the play behaviors of children.

Arousal-seeking is the third theoretical conception of play. It conceives of play as caused by the need to generate interactions with the environment or self that elevates arousal (level of interest or stimulation) toward the optimal for the individual child. It assumes that stimuli vary in their capacity to arouse, that there is a need for optimal arousal, that movement toward optimal arousal is pleasant, and that the organism learns the behaviors that result in that feeling and vice versa.

Finally, *competence/effectance,* the fourth theory, conceives of play as caused by a need to produce effects in the environment. Such effects demonstrate competence and result in feelings of effectance. This theory assumes that demonstrations of competence lead to feelings of effectance, that effectance is pleasant, and that effectance increases the probability of competence.

Taken together, these four theories carry considerable implications for the design of playspaces. Developmentalism implies that playspaces should provide for wide ranges of developmental diversity in motoric, intellectual, and social functioning. Learning theory implies that reinforcement devices, positive experiences, feedback, novelty, and change should also be incorporated in playspaces. Arousal-seeking theory implies that utilitarian equipment, equipment capable of being changed and restructured by children to meet their needs for optimal arousal, would be appropriate. Competence/effectance theory implies that children need opportunities to change and restructure their play environments.

Developmentally Appropriate Equipment

Preschool and primary school teachers are often hard pressed to provide equipment which can accomodate the wide ranges of skillfulness and readiness within their children. More often than not, commercially available equipment is suited for use by a narrow, and usually highly skilled range of children. Rubber utility balls are often so heavy they lie unused in nursery schools. Hoop targets are often permanently placed at so high a level that only intermediate school children can use them. Rackets, bats, and paddles tend to be so long and heavy that children abandon them or use them for other purposes than gross motor play. Recent research indicates that lightweight striking, throwing, and kicking equipment can encourage more mature and effecient gross motor performances and can foster faster gross motor learning than was thought possible for children exposed to more traditional equipment (Halverson, 1966).

Three guidelines may provide some help in providing adequately for wide ranges of skillfulness and readiness. *Grouping pieces of equipment that have the same form, but which vary in size* provides one solution. Figures 7-1 through 7-5 provide illustrations of this principle.

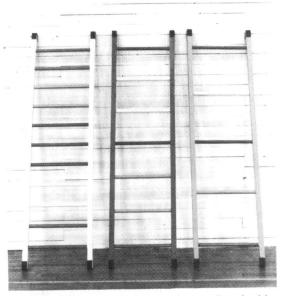

Figure 7-1. Three vertical ladders leaning against a wall, each with rungs a different distance apart.

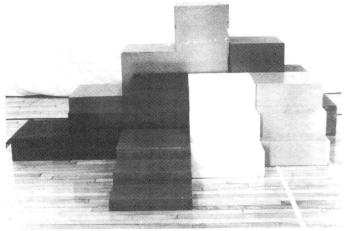

Figure 7-2. Six staircases, each with different height and depth stairs.

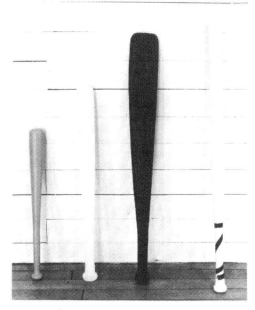

Figure 7-3. Four different length and width plastic bats.

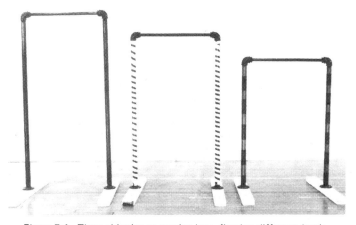

Figure 7-4. Three chinning or turning bars, fixed at different levels.

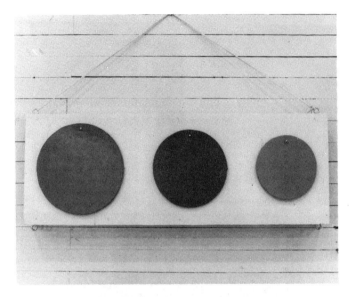

Figure 7-5. Three disc kicking or throwing targets of different sizes which will "buzz" when struck.

A second way of providing for extensive individual differences is to *select equipment that children can adjust to accommodate their own developmental levels.* For example:

1. A metal hoop throwing target, fixed on a collapsible stand, and held in place by a wing bolt that children can adjust to raise or lower the hoop.
2. A ball suspended on sashcord and tied with a hangman's noose so that the child can raise or lower the ball (see Figure 7-6).
3. A wand supported by vertical standards which children can raise or lower before jumping or leaping over (see Figure 7-7).
4. A batting-*t* fitted with a length of rubber tubing which a child may raise or lower to change the height of a supported ball (see Figure 7-8).

5. A sliding board that children can tilt to any inclination before climbing or sliding down.
6. A support and an adjustable incline, down which balls can rolled before being struck or caught (see Figure 7-9).
7. A lightweight ball supported at various levels by an exhaust vacuum cleaner air jet channeled through a crevice tool; all housed in a wooden box (see Figure 7-10).

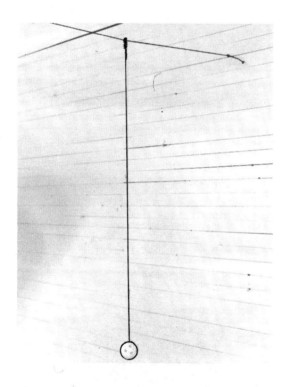

Figure 7-6. A ball suspended on sashcord and tied with a hangman's noose which may be raised or lowered.

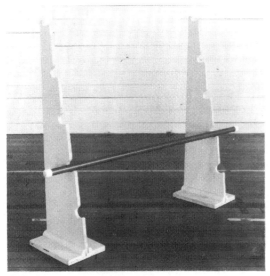

Figure 7-7. A wand supported by vertical standards which children can raise or lower before jumping or leaping over.

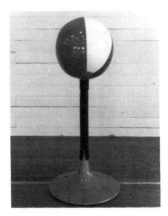

Figure 7-8. A batting-*t* fixed with a length of rubber tubing which a child may raise or lower to change the height of a supported ball.

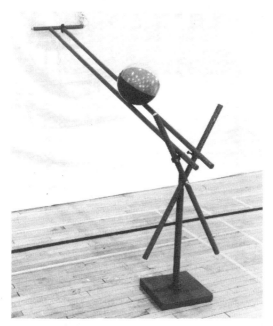

Figure 7-9. A support and an adjustable incline, down which balls can be rolled before being struck or caught.

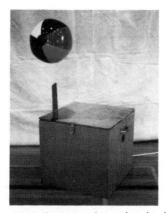

Figure 7-10. A lightweight ball supported at various levels by an exhaust vacuum cleaner air jet channeled through a crevice tool; all housed in a wooden box.

A third way of providing for differences is to *give children single pieces of equipment which, by their very structure, accommodate wide ranges of developmental levels.* For example:

1. A walking board which is very wide at one end and increasingly more narrow toward the other end (see Figure 7-11).
2. A vertical knotted rope which children can climb only as high as they wish.
3. A horizontal ladder with increasingly wider-spaced rungs at one end and narrowly spaced rungs at the other end.

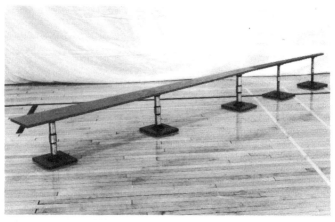

Figure 7-11. A walking board which is very wide at one end and increasingly more narrow toward the other end.

Change and Variety in Playspaces

An environment to which new pieces of equipment and equipment groups are added and well-used ones are eliminated or reconstructed frequently is also desirable in light of the four theoretical positions regarding play discussed earlier. As a result, equipment which is mobile is far preferable to that which is permanently embedded in walls, floors, or the ground. This does not imply, of course, that a swing frame or a climbing tower are undesirable. By attaching new items to them or placing other equipment around them, their ability to stimulate new movement experiences becomes enormous—and in this sense, they are exceptions. Traditional slides, teeter-totters, and merry-go-rounds do not lend themselves to change and variety, however, and are, therefore, of comparatively limited value.

Children can do much to build their environment to meet their own complexity requirements if the apparatus presented them can be reconstructed and manipulated by them. Currently, much apparatus that is commercially available allows children to manipulate themselves by swinging and whirling. And children give their sustained attention and respond most to equipment they can manipulate.

The most desirable movement equipment, then, should be utilitarian in the sense that it can be reorganized or placed within a variety of apparatus configurations by the child to encourage many movement possibilities. For example, apparatus such as aluminum trestles and platforms work well. This equipment may be rearranged by children or adults to provide the youngsters with many climbing and balancing tasks. It may also be arranged with other equipment such as ropes, balls, and cargo net to stimulate more movements. Equipment such as spring-supported animals and teeter-totters seems relatively nonutilitarian by comparison.

Locked and ample storage space should be provided which takes into account the height and strength of the preschooler or primary school child. A combination climbing tower-storage shed which houses large apparatus, small vehicles, and containers for small apparatus will facilitate the construction and use of an outdoor environment. Adults and children will be able to spend less time taking equipment from and returning it to storage. Small equipment should be arranged on readily accessible shelves or stored in boxes that children can move freely. Frequently, such storage is unavailable—and then serious limits are placed on change, variety, and projectile-associated movement opportunities.

Whether a play area has one or a variety of surfaces may also influence the variety of movement opportunities provided children. Tanbark, sand, sawdust, or rubber matting lying below climbing apparatus encourages safe climbing, swinging, and hanging. Cement and asphalt encourage vehicular play and ball bouncing, but they discourage climbing, hanging, and swinging. Running, rolling, skipping, galloping, hopping, jumping, and balancing are easier on soil, turf, and synthetic turf surfaces. Similarly, gravel, sand, water, and uneven or inclined surfaces encourage additional unique ways of moving.

The amount of equipment provided children in playspaces also influences their behavior. In an early study, Johnson (1935) found that more extensively equipped playgrounds are associated with greater bodily exercise levels and less undesirable social behavior, while less extensively equipped playgrounds spawn less bodily exercise, less play with materials, and more social contacts and social conflicts. Wade (1970), on the other hand, also studying preschool children, more recently found that lesser or more equipment had very little influence on the telemetered activity levels of 16 kindergarten children. Our very few research results thus tend to conflict with each other.

Research findings regarding the use of playspaces which do not change over time are also equivocal. Wuellner (1969) investigated the differences between the movement patterns of 4- and 5-year-old children over successive play sessions before and after new objects were introduced. Among other findings, Wuellner noted that activity—distance moved—generally decreased over successive sessions. On the other hand, Karlsson (1970) investigated the frequency of vertical movement during play by 4- and 5-year-old children. It was expected that repeated exposures would lead to increasing ability to cope with the apparatus, and that the children's height preference would increase. This did not happen either for any one type of apparatus or overall. The failure to find trends suggested that the five play sessions may have represented a cross-sectional sample of play rather than the longitudinal one which Karlsson anticipated, since it is a common observation that children learn to climb higher with exposure. It remains for researchers to determine to what extent boredom, undesirable social behavior, activity levels, social behavior, and skill development are influenced by changing and static environments.

At present, most movement environments encourage climbing, hanging, and swinging. They devote very little attention to other types of gross and fine motor behavior such as striking, catching, throwing, kicking, balancing, rolling objects, rolling oneself, zipping, lacing, buttoning, cutting, locking, latching, snapping, buckling, stacking, fitting, pushing and pulling, dancing, and swimming. Perhaps attention needs to be paid to incorporating greater varieties of movement into playspaces. If children are to seize upon critical learning periods and build up a strong repertoire of movement experiences (upon which, later, more complex dance, sports, and work skills can be built), variety must be a part of playspaces.

Incorporating Reinforcement into the Environment

In recent years, behavior modification techniques have been used extensively to produce rapid and relevant changes in the academic, motor, and social behavior of a variety of children in numerous situations. By programming materials and carefully managing the consequences of appropriate and inappropriate behavior, behavioral deficits and deviances have been reduced and training of normal and handicapped children has been accelerated with remarkable efficiency and success. As a result both standard education and remedial and therapeutic practices increasingly are incorporating procedures and principles derived from research in behavior modification.

Rarely, however, have we invaded playspaces with ideas designed to lead children to make responses which increase their skillfulness. It would seem similar programming and contingency management procedures also should and could be applied beneficially to the environment of free play. The power of nonverbal reinforcing agents incorporated into the apparatus included on playspaces has not been explored. It is conceivable

the novelty of lights, buzzers, horns, bells, color, and movement would provide potentially powerful reinforcement for
desirable movement performances. For example, children may
be more likely to throw at a metal target since it makes considerable noise when hit. Figures 7-12 through 7-15 provide illustrations of devices which reinforce desirable movement responses.

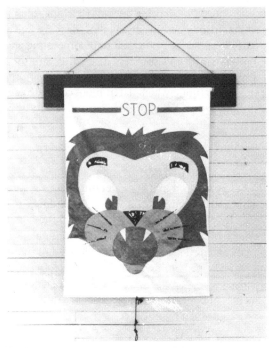

Figure 7-12. A windowshade on which a colorful lion is painted which
will roll up if hit with a tennis or yarn ball thrown with sufficient force.

Evaluative Devices and Feedback

Environmental design techniques can also encourage children to
assess their own skillfulness more realistically. By painting each
of the rungs of a rope ladder a different color, a teacher may help

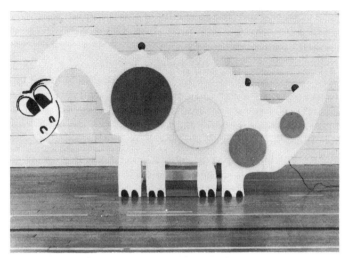

Figure 7-13. A plywood dragon on which are placed four different-sized circular targets. When hit, the targets trigger lightning or matching colored bulbs.

children to evaluate, and communicate to others, their own ability to negotiate the ladder. The same is true when several parallel lines of different colors are placed various distances from targets. Using timing devices that involve the clock arm turning through various simply numbered or differently colored areas on the clock face, while a child performs any variety of movement tasks, is still another example. These techniques may be especially significant considering the rapid changes in growth and skillfulness associated with the preschool and primary school years—and if one organizes the stimuli around the theories of play discussed previously.

Organization of the Playspace

The shape, size, and division of the playspace, and the placement of apparatus and hard surface pathways in the playspace all influence the movement behavior of children (Kritchevsky & Prescott,

1969). For example, the popularity of equipment and apparatus, as well as the physical activity level of children in a playspace, may well be influenced by the positioning of apparatus in the environment. In a study by Witt and Gramza (1970), a large and small trestle were interchanged between center and corner positions in a series of play sessions and the frequency with which preschool children used the trestles in each position was recorded. Three out of four groups of children tested used the trestle more when it was in the center position than when it was placed in the corner. Not only may centrally located equipment, surrounded by open space, enjoy more popularity than apparatus placed in corners, in isolated areas, or around the edge of playspaces; but it is also conceivable that different apparatus placement config-

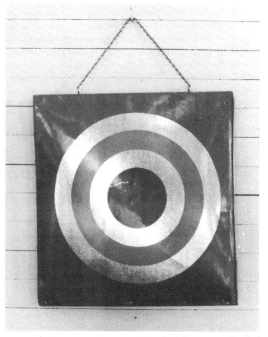

Figure 7-14. A sheet metal target painted with concentric circles.

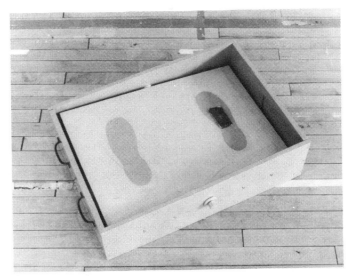

Figure 7-15. A stabilometer which "buzzes" when a child causes it to remain in balance.

urations (for example, along one side of the environment, all grouped in one corner, placed in separate corners) may differentially influence the popularity of individual pieces of apparatus as well as the general activity level within the environment. Apparatus placed near entrance ways to playspaces will probably enjoy more initial attention than those placed farther away. It is conceivable that moving an unpopular piece of apparatus between two pieces which are in the same movement environment, but are very popular, can change the degree of use of the unpopular apparatus. Divisions of movement environments caused by fencing and surfacing techniques can create isolated areas ideal for projectile activities such as striking, throwing, kicking, and catching.

The relationship of apparatus placement to open space also deserves attention. An open, unobstructed outdoor area, intended to encourage running, sliding, galloping, striking, and balancing, may not be effectively used if children travel across that open area to get from one piece of apparatus to another. Apparatus placed to one side of a large area may help to encourage free locomotor and manipulative activity in the remaining space.

Similarly, the use of hard surface pathways and fence barriers has an impact on how children will use the play environment. If pathways are laid between large pieces of apparatus, children riding vehicles may collide with children traveling from one piece of apparatus to another. Perhaps hard surface pathways should surround a play environment rather than run through it. Shelves, boxes, pianos, walls, partitions, and fences can well influence the speed with which children travel through play environments and which equipment will be the most focal and popular, as well as the general activity level in the environment.

Apparatus can be designed and ordered to take into account desirable ways of having children travel through the movement environment or across a complex play structure. Ramps leading down from structures, cargo nets and ropes connecting different pieces of apparatus, stairways, and sliding poles all provide avenues of entrance, exit, and transit through the environment. These should be carefully thought through.

Socialization in the Playspace

It seems that certain types of apparatus stimulate social interaction more than other types. For example, tire swings, manipulative cubes, interactive rope-pole climbers, cargo nets, and apparatus with built-in directional pathways that converge would all cause more social interaction than apparatus such as a batting-*t* or a manipulative board.

Van Alstyne (1932), studying choice and use of play materials by preschool children, reported that over 50 percent of children at all ages played alone when playing with materials. She also noted that older children played more cooperatively and were more social. Johnson (1935) concluded that as the amount of play equipment decreased, the amount of aggressive behavior and social interaction increased among preschool children. Barker (1930) studied the social-material activities of young children and found that as age increased, the number of social contacts increased while the number of activities engaged in decreased.

Evaluation Techniques

Playgrounds, once designed, should be evaluated. A number of observational techniques can provide enormous information about the frequency, duration, and nature of movements children demonstrate within a planned play environment. Numerous research investigations have employed several of these techniques. Dow (1933) charted subject movement in a study of the reactions of children to the presence or absence of playground equipment. The observer, stationed so that all four experimental areas were in view, traced onto scaled plans of the proper area the movement of a subject from point to point for 1-minute intervals and made a running descriptive account at the same time. Swinton (1934) used a time-lapse camera mounted on a roof to record simultaneously the movement of several subjects on a playground. The activity of a group of 5-year-old children for 1 hour was filmed using 2-second intervals between pictures. The movement paths of each child were traced onto pictures of the playground, 1 minute of film being recorded on each picture, to reveal the interest value of the equipment, the amount and character of physical activity, and social behavior.

In an attempt to objectify the observations and to improve their reliability further, workers at the University of Illinois developed a new method to record and analyze the movement of children at play (Herron & Frobish, 1969; Wuellner, 1969; Wuellner, Witt & Herron, 1970). This method used a camera mounted above a play area which automatically takes pictures at preset intervals. A fisheye lens enables the total play area to be within the field of view. The film is projected onto a grid and the coordinates describing the location of each apparatus area and each subject are recorded from a frame-by-frame inspection. Computer analysis of these coordinates gives a record of each child's activity as well as of his interactions with the other players and the equipment.

Wade (1968) studied the free-play patterns of elementary school children in playground equipment areas by photographing each area and its immediate environs once per minute, with recorded narration of observable play patterns. His data analysis used modern techniques which attempted to compare play patterns according to apparatus categories, day observed, and the socioeconomic level of the child. His analysis considered visit time and percent of time on various apparatus types. He also made use of telemetry to monitor activity levels of children.

In schools, teachers have a number of techniques available which they may use to monitor the effects and influences of environment on children. These are *event recording, duration recording, Placheck, time sampling, interval recording,* and *continuous recording* (Cooper, 1974; Hall, 1971); and they can provide an objective basis on which to reconstruct a play environment. *Event recording* involves making a frequency count of a specific movement behavior demonstrated during a defined period of time. For example, a teacher could find out the number of times children demonstrate striking behaviors within a given movement environment. If a teacher uses *duration recording,* recording elapsed time spent performing a given movement behavior during a specified length of time, he or she would find out, for example, how much time a piece of climbing apparatus is used by children in a group.

Placheck (Planned Activity Check) involves the teacher's counting as quickly as possible at given intervals (say, each 10-minute mark during a 30-minute period), how many children are engaged in a specific movement behavior as well as the total number of children present in the movement environment. The number of children performing, divided by the number present, all multiplied by 100, will provide the percent of those engaged in the movement behavior at particular times during an activity period. *Interval recording* is used to measure the occurrence or nonoccurrence of behavior within specified intervals. *Time sampling* is used to measure the occurence or nonoccurrence of behavior at the end of specified time intervals. *Continuous recording* involves the production of a written record or narrative for a specified time period of individual or group behaviors.

Conclusion

A good portion of young children's life experience may be shaped by the environment in which they find themselves. Researchers have just begun to ask and answer questions about what play behavior to expect when specific equipment and equipment configurations are presented to children, which of these apparatus children prefer and use most frequently, and which need to be changed to encourage high interest and activity. These and similar questions eventually will be answered. Until then, perhaps the practitioner—armed with the four theories of play discussed earlier, his or her intuitions about how environmental variables influence play behavior, and observational techniques which allow him to evaluate objectively what is happening in a playspace—may even more meaningfully approach the design, construction, and reconstruction of playspaces for children.

REFERENCES

Barker, M. A. Technique for studying the social-material activities of young children. New York: Columbia University Press (Child Development Monograph No. 3), 1930.

Cooper, J. O. *Measurement and Analysis of Behavioral Techniques.* Columbus: Merrill, 1974.

Dow, M. Playground behavior differentiating artistic from nonartistic children. *Psychological Monographs,* 1933, *45,* 82-94.

Ellis, M. J. Play and its theories re-examined. *Parks and Recreation,* August, 1971, 51-55, 89-90.

Ellis, M. J. The rational design of playgrounds. *Educational Product Report,* 1970, *3,* 3-6.

Hall, R. V. *Managing Behavior.* Lawrence, Kans.: H. & H. Enterprises, 1971.

Halverson, L. E. Development of motor patterns in young children. *Quest,* Monograph 6, 1966, 44-53.

Herron, R. E., & Frobish, M. J. Computer analysis and display of movement patterns. *Journal of Experimental Child Psychology,* 1969, *8,* 40-44.

Johnson, M. W. The effect on behavior of variation in the amount of play equipment. *Child Development,* 1935, *6* (1), 56-68.

Karlsson, K. A. Height preferences of young children at play. Unpublished master's thesis, University of Illinois, 1970.

Kritchevsky, S., & Prescott, E. *Planning Environments for Young Children.* Washington, D. C.: National Association for the Education of Young Children, 1969.

Swinton, R. S. Analysis of child behavior by intermittent photography. *Child Development,* 1934, *5,* 292-293.

Van Alstyne, D. *Play Behavior and Choice of Play Materials of Preschool Children.* Chicago: University of Chicago Press, 1932.

Wade, G. R. Biorhythms in children during free play. Unpublished Ph.D. dissertation, University of Illinois at Urbana-Champaign, 1970.

Wade, G. R. A study of free-play patterns of elementary school-age children in playground equipment areas. Unpublished master's thesis, Pennsylvania State University, 1968.

Witt, P. A., & Gramza, A. F. Position effects in play equipment preferences of nursery school children. *Perceptual & Motor Skills,* 1970, *31,* 431-434.

Wuellner, L. A. A method to investigate the movement patterns of children. Unpublished master's thesis, University of Illinois, 1969.

Wuellner, L. A. The present status of research on playgrounds. *Educational Product Review*, 1970, *3*, 8-12.

Wuellner, L. A., Witt, P. A., & Herron, R. E. A method to investigate the movement patterns of children. Proceedings of the Second International Congress of Sport Psychology, 1970.

8

Developmental Task Analysis: The Design of Movement Experiences and Evaluation of Motor Development Status

JACQUELINE HERKOWITZ

Many task and environmental variables figure prominently in efforts to acquire and perform motor skills. A child does not *just strike a ball.* Striking a ball involves innumerable variables acting in concert. A child strikes a certain sized ball, a certain weight ball, a ball that has certain speed and trajectory characteristics. And if he is to grow more skilled, he must learn to deal with such variables at increasingly complex levels; he must learn to hit increasingly smaller balls, increasingly faster balls, and balls which have trajectories that are increasingly less predictable. If an instructor is to be successful in helping a child, he must be able to identify such task and environmental variables, understand their interactive influences on performance, manipulate these variables to provide developmentally appropriate and challenging movement experiences, and evaluate the effect of his manipulations on performance. This discussion is designed to assist the instructor in the performance of these tasks.

Developmental Task Analysis may be thought of either as a testing device which assesses the motor developmental status of children or as an instructional approach which involves the design of sequentially ordered motor experiences and the identification of variables which limit motor skill acquisition. It involves two components: (1) *General Task Analysis* (GTA), and (2) *Specific Task Analysis* (STA), which is based upon GTA. GTAs involve defining any and all task and environmental factors which influence the movement behavior of children in a general motor category (such as striking, throwing, catching, jumping, kicking, running, and climbing), either alone or in combination. For example, in Table 8-1, a GTA for striking behavior is provided which identifies seven factors influencing any striking behavior regardless of the person performing or the specific nature of the task being performed. Certainly, far more than seven could be identified, but for the purposes of this example, seven will suffice. The degree to which striking tasks involve factors on simple or complex levels is indicated by the *levels* section of the GTA. The levels imply that not all conditions of the same factor are equatable. That is, children encountering factors at simple levels would find those tasks easier to perform than tasks involving the same factors at more complex levels. The level within each factor varies depending upon the demands of the particular task being described. For instance, in Table 8-1, the first factor identified is the *size of object to be struck*. The levels are broadly classified as large, medium, and small, indicating that in this one factor, by decreasing the size of the object being struck we may contribute to the complexity of the task and, perhaps, the difficulty experienced by children who respond to the task.

Any particular striking behavior may be termed a *profile*. Two profiles are delineated in Table 8-1: one relatively simple, and the other relatively complex. The simple profile represents a child striking a large, light, stationary ball with his hand, when the ball is positioned to his favored side and he is standing next to it. The relatively complex profile represents a child striking a small, light ball, which is moving at a fast speed, rebounding off the ground, with a fairly long implement, when the ball is traveling to his nonfavored side, and he must make considerable locomotor adjustments before he can reach the ball. The first profile might represent a child's first efforts to hit a beach ball suspended on a string. The second profile might well describe a tennis player making a backhand stroke during a game. Essentially, such profiles are movement behaviors involving certain delineated factors, considered at unique levels.

Once one becomes familiar with factors that influence behavior in a general motor category, such as were shown in Table 8-1,

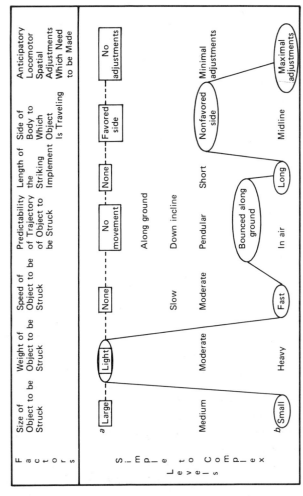

Table 8-1. General Task Analysis for Striking Behavior

aProfile of a GTA for a relatively simple striking task (dotted line).
bProfile of a GTA for a relatively complex striking task (solid line).

one may begin to examine how these factors influence performance in specific tasks. Such an examination is termed an STA, and represents the second component of Developmental Task Analysis.

STAs are formed by inventing activities that incorporate certain factors from the GTA that we wish to view in combination across all their levels. An example of a STA involving striking is illustrated in Figure 8-1. In this STA three factors have been chosen from the GTA for examination: the size of the object to be struck, length of the striking implement, and predictability of the trajectory of the object to be struck. The child's task is to strike three of four balls out of a goal area measuring 5 by 3 yards. The progressive developmental expectations are that the children should perform this task with increasingly smaller sized balls, with implements that are increasingly longer, and with balls whose trajectories are increasingly less predictable. All three factors carry with them *level designations,* much as was the case in GTAs. The only difference is that the level designations in the STA become far more specific and defined than they are in a GTA. Each level within each factor in the STA is translated into designated items of equipment and task specifications. In factor one, the size of the ball varies from 12 inches to approximately 2 inches in diameter. Factor two, length of the implement, includes the hand, ping pong paddle, dowel rod, and a plastic bat. Factor three, predictability of the trajectory, includes the ball traveling along the ground with no bounce, bounced along the ground and traveling through the air. Levels within each factor move from simple to complex, making the task and subsequent progressions more difficult for the child to master.

Profiles of performance for a STA are conceived in much the same manner as is the case for the GTA. The only difference is that the level designations become more concretely defined. Varied profiles can be identified within the STA by changing the levels of each factor. Thus, the teacher or evaluator is at liberty to test different children at different levels of complexity by selecting certain profiles for evaluation of specific children.

Task:
Striking

Child's Task:
To strike approximately 3 of 4 balls out of a goal area which is 5 yards by 3 yards.

Activity:
"Keep-Out"

The child should be able to do this for:

Equipment:
12" beach ball
9" beach ball
4" wiffle ball
tennis ball
ping pong paddle
18" dowel rod
36" plastic bat

1. Increasingly smaller sized balls.
2. Implements that are increasingly longer in length.
3. Balls whose trajectories are increasingly less predictable.

Factors Influencing Student Performance			
	Size of Ball	Length of Striking Implement	Predictability of the Trajectory of the Ball
S i m p l e **Levels of Complex** t o C o m p l e x	*S1* 12" beach ball	*L1* hand	*P1* along ground (no bounce)
	S2 9" beach ball	*L2* ping pong paddle	*P2* bounced along ground
	S3 4" wiffle ball	*L3* 18" dowel rod (wooden)	*P3* aerial ball
	S4 tennis ball	*L4* 36" plastic bat	

Figure 8-1. Specific Task Analysis for striking.

STAs can be used to place a child along a developmental continuum with regard to possible STA profiles. This is done through the use of a *grid evaluation* (see Figure 8-2). This composite chart displays all possible profiles in the form of "cells." When a child performs a specific profile, the date of accomplishment is recorded in the appropriate cell. This way, the rate and direction of a child's progress can be examined. Factors providing the child with the greatest difficulty may be defined and dealt with by the teacher. If groups of children appear to be having difficulty with a factor or combination of factors, the teacher can concentrate on that problem. It is conceivable that patterns of profile accomplishment could eventually even help to distinguish various groups of children (such as the mentally handicapped or learning disabled). Similarly, teachers can use the concepts of STA and GTA to guide and design the sequencing of movement experiences for children.

Assessment											
$P1^a$				$P2$				$P3$			
$L1^b$	$L2$	$L3$	$L4$	$L1$	$L2$	$L3$	$L4$	$L1$	$L2$	$L3$	$L4$

	$L1^b$	$L2$	$L3$	$L4$	$L1$	$L2$	$L3$	$L4$	$L1$	$L2$	$L3$	$L4$
$S1^c$												
$S2$												
$S3$												
$S4$												

aP1	along ground with no bounce	bL1	hand	cS1	12" beach ball
P2	bounced along ground	L2	ping pong paddle	S2	9" beach ball
P3	aerial ball	L3	18" wooden dowel rod	S3	4" wiffle ball
		L4	36" plastic bat	S4	tennis ball

Figure 8-2. Grid evaluation for striking Specific Task Analysis.

Perhaps one of the most meaningful strengths of Developmental Task Analysis is its lack of emphasis on age-appropriate behaviors. A 6-year-old does not have to perform certain prescribed skills. Instead, the major thrust is to place children along developmental continua, with little concern for what is, in fact, age-appropriate. Little research data are available to provide such insights today. Too much emphasis on age-appropriate behavior in reading and mathematics in the past has only frustrated teachers and parents. Developmental Task Analysis encourages those interested in the movement behavior of children to acknowledge the complexity of motor performance, and make use of that knowledge in designing movement experiences and evaluating developmental status. Perhaps the greatest weakness is that it requires, as an assessment device, extensive administration time, and considerable record keeping. Wall charts and computerized record keeping can do much, however, to alleviate some of these constraints.

Developmental Task Analysis also confronts researchers with a myriad of questions regarding the relationship of task and environment variables and their influence on performance. At the present time, researchers have answered few of the questions that would support the logic demonstrated in intuitively derived GTAs and STAs. Until they do, intuition will have to continue to provide the matrix around which this technique will develop. Many studies have been undertaken to describe the components underlying motor performance (Cumbee 1954; Fleishman, 1958; Jackson, 1971; McCloy, 1956; Rarick, 1937; Rarick & Dobbins, 1975). These studies have sought to extract common factor variances from large sets of physical performance measures in order to identify these basic motor properties (Cumbee, 1954). While this approach has contributed significantly to broadening the scientific understanding of motor abilities, it has provided little of functional value to the practitioner who must deal with the day-to-day problems of helping children acquire striking, catching, throwing, jumping, kicking, running, and climbing skills. More recent perceptual investigations of children's abilities to deal with moving projectiles (Adams & Creamer, 1962; Gallahue, 1968;

Herkowitz, 1972; Ridenour, 1974; Williams, 1968) appear to provide the beginnings of what may well become an empirical basis for Developmental Task Analysis.

The following representative GTAs (Tables 8-2 through 8-7) and STAs (Figures 8-3 through 8-14) for the fundamental motor patterns of catching, jumping, running, throwing, kicking, and climbing, are provided to facilitate the reader's use of the Developmental Task Analysis technique.

Table 8-2. General Task Analysis for Catching Behavior

Factors	Weight of Object to be Caught	Speed of Catcher's Movement Prior To Catch	Direction in Which Catcher Must Move Prior to Catch	Size of Object Being Caught	Speed of Object to be Caught	Level Object Is Traveling to with Regard to Catcher	Length of Extension Used to Catch With
Simplest to Complex Levels	Moderate	No movement	Forward	Moderate	No movement	Chest level	None
		Slow			Slow	Above head slightly	
	Light		Sideward	Large		Waist level	Moderate
	Moderate	Moderate			Moderate	Knee level	
	Heavy	Fast	Backward	Small	Fast	Foot level	Long

Table 8-3. General Task Analysis for Jumping Behavior

Factors / Levels of Complexity	Size of the Takeoff Surface	Size of the Surface to be Landed On	Distance to be Traversed in the Jump	Speed of the Jump Required	Amount of Momentum Built Prior to Takeoff	Direction of the Jump	Level to be Jumped To
	Large	Large	Short	Slow	Little	Forward	Same
	Moderate	Moderate	Moderate	Moderate	Moderate	Sideward	Low
	Small	Small	Long	Fast	Great	Backward	High

Table 8-4. General Task Analysis for Running Behavior

Factors	Speed Required	Amount of Time Run Must be Sustained	Direction Of the Run	Inclination of the Running Surface	With Equipment of Various Sizes	With Equipment of Various Weights	Changes of Direction Required
	Moderate	Short	Forward	None	Small	Light	None
				Slight upward incline			
	Slow	Moderate	Backward	Slight downward incline	Moderate	Moderate	Few
				Steep upward incline			
	Fast	Long	Sideward	Steep downward incline	Large	Heavy	Many

Simple to Complex Levels

Table 8-5. General Task Analysis for Throwing Behavior

	Size of the Object Being Thrown	Distance Object Must be Thrown	Weight of the Object Being Thrown	Accuracy Required of the Throw	Speed at Which Target Being Thrown At Is Moving	Acceleration & Deceleration Characteristics of the Target Being Thrown At	Direction in Which Target Being Thrown At Is Moving
Simple	Small	Short	Moderately light	None	Stationary	No movement	No movement
			Moderately heavy	Little	Slow	Steady speed	Left to right of thrower
	Medium	Medium					Right to left of thrower
			Light	Moderate	Moderate	Decelerating	Toward thrower
Complex	Large	Long	Heavy	Much	Fast	Accelerating	Away from thrower

Table 8-6. General Task Analysis for Kicking Behavior

Factors	Direction Object is Traveling in With Regard to Receiver	Size of Object Being Kicked	Speed With Which Ball Is Traveling Prior to the Kick	Portion of the Foot Which Must Be Used to Contact the Ball	Anticipatory Locomotor Spatial Adjustments Which Need to be Made Prior to the Kick	Direction in Which Kicker Must Move Prior to Kick
Simple to Complex Levels	Favored side	Moderate	Slow	Toe	No adjustments	No movement
				Inside edge		
	Midline	Large	Moderate	Outside edge	Minimal adjustments	Forward
				Instep		Sideward
	Nonfavored side	Small	Fast	Heel	Maximal adjustments	Backward

Table 8-7. General Task Analysis for Climbing Behavior

	Distance That Must be Traversed	Number of Body Parts That May be Used	Angle At Which Person Must Climb	Speed At Which Person Must Climb	Stability of Climbing Apparatus	Level to Which Person Must Climb	Direction In Which Person Must Climb
	Short	Many	None	Slow	Rigid	Low	Forward
Simple to Complex Levels	Moderate	Some	Small	Moderate		Moderate	Sideward
	Long	Few	Great	Fast	Unstable	High	Backward

Task:
Climbing

Activity:
"Climb-the-Plank"

Equipment:
9' x 2' x 3/4" board
12' rope
8' high stall bars with
    6" distances between
    the rungs

Child's Task:
To climb up and down an inclined
board which is 9' long and 2' wide,
without touching hands to the board.

The child should be able to do this for:

1. Increasingly more steep inclinations.
2. Moving forward before moving backward.
3. Climbing with the assistance of a
   free-hanging rope before climbing
   without the assistance of such a rope.

Factors Influencing Student Performance			
	Steepness of Incline	Direction	Assistance
Simple Level to Complex	S1 1st or 2nd rung	D1 upward	A1 use of free-hanging rope
	S2 3rd or 4th rung	D2 downward	A2 no use of free-hanging rope
	S3 5th or 6th rung		
	S4 7th or 8th rung		
	S5 9th or 10th rung		
	S6 11th or 12th rung		
	S7 13th or 14th rung		
	S8 15th or 16th rung		

Figure 8-3. Specific Task Analysis for climbing.

Assessment				
	D1		D2	
	A1	A2	A1	A2
S1				
S2				
S3				
S4				
S5				
S6				
S7				
S8				

S1 1st and 2nd rung   D1 Upward   A1 Use of Rope
S2 3rd and 4th rung   D2 Downward   A2 No Use of Rope
S3 5th and 6th rung
S4 7th and 8th rung
S5 9th and 10th rung
S6 11th and 12th rung
S7 13th and 14th rung
S8 15th and 16th rung

Figure 8-4. Grid evaluation for climbing Specific Task Analysis.

Task:
Jumping

Activity:
"Jump For
 Speed"

Equipment:
1 yard pieces
of rope or
chalk lines

Child's Task:
To repeatedly jump across a 1 yard piece
of rope or chalked line, without touching
it. Do this as many times as possible in 15
seconds. A jump is defined as a movement
involving a 2 foot take-off and a 2 foot landing.

The child should be able to jump:

1. At increasingly greater speeds.
2. Sideward before foward-backward.

Factors Influencing Student Performance		
	Direction of Jump	Number of Jumps Completed in 15 Seconds
S i m p l e **L e v e l s** **C o m p l e x**	*D1* sideward	*J1* 1
	D2 forward-backward	*J2* 2
		J3 3
		J4 4
		J5 5
		J6 7
		J7 10
		J8 15
		J9 20

Figure 8-5. Specific Task Analysis for jumping.

Assessment		
	D1	*D2*
J1		
J2		
J3		
J4		
J5		
J6		
J7		
J8		
J9		

D1 sideward

D2 forward-backward

J1 1 jump
J2 2 jumps
J3 3 jumps
J4 4 jumps
J5 5 jumps
J6 7 jumps
J7 10 jumps
J8 15 jumps
J9 20 jumps

Figure 8-6. Grid for jumping Specific Task Analysis.

Task:
Running

Activity:
"Run-Around"

Equipment:
12 12"-high cone markers
running course which is
  50 yards x 15 yards
  with 6 gates made of
  2 cone markers set 1
  yard apart and placed
  alternately on the side-
  lines to form a zig-zag
  course

Child's Task
To run through an obstacle course
as quickly as possible.

The child should be able to complete the
course:

1. Carrying increasingly heavier weights
   in each hand.
2. At increasingly faster speeds.
3. Demonstrating increasing numbers
   of direction changes.

Factors Influencing Student Performance			
	Weights Being Carried in Each Hand	Speed of the Run	Number of Gates That Have to be Traversed in Sequence
S	*W1* no weights	*S1* 40 sec. or more	*G1* gates 1, 2
i			
m			
p		*S2* 39.9-30 sec.	
l			
L e	*W2* 2 lb. weights		
e		*S3* 29.9-20 sec.	
v t			
e o			*G2* gates 1, 2, 3, 4
l		*S4* 19.9-15 sec.	
s C	*W3* 5 lb. weights		
o		*S5* 14.9-10 sec.	
m			
p	*W4* 8 lb. weights	*S6* 9.9 sec. or less	*G3* gates 1, 2, 3, 4, 5, 6
l e			
x			

Figure 8-7. Specific Task Analysis for running.

Assessment											
W1			W2			W3			W4		
G1	G2	G3	G1	G2	G3	G1	G2	G3	G1	G2	G3
S1											
S2											
S3											
S4											
S5											
S6											

S1 40 sec. or more   *W1* no weights   *G1* gates 1, 2
S2 39.9-30 sec.   *W2* 2 lb. weights   *G2* gates 1, 2, 3, 4
S3 29.9-20 sec.   *W3* 5 lb. weights   *G3* gates 1, 2, 3, 4, 5, 6
S4 19.9-15 sec.   *W4* 8 lb. weights
S5 14.9-10 sec.
S6 9.9 sec. or less

Figure 8-8. Grid evaluation for running Specific Task Analysis.

Task:
Throwing

Child's Task:
To throw at least 1 out of 5 tennis balls overhand so that it hits a beach ball hanging from a 6' cord which is swinging in a side to side pendular trajectory in front of the thrower.

Activity:
"Hit-The-Pendulum"

Equipment:
3 beach balls suspended on 6 foot cords, 12", 8", and 4" in diameter
tape marks on floor 9', 18', and 24' from the target

The child should be able to do this for:
1. Ball targets which are increasingly smaller.
2. Distances that are increasingly farther from the target.
3. Targets which are moving at increasingly greater ranges of motion.

Factors Influencing Student Performance				
		Size of The Target	Distance	Range of Motion of the Pendulum
S i m p l e	S1	12" beach ball	D1 9'	R1 3' arc
L e v e l s t o	S2	8" beach ball	D2 18'	R2 5' arc
C o m p l e x	S3	4" beach ball	D3 24'	R3 7' arc

Figure 8-9. Specific Task Analysis for Throwing.

Assessment								
D1			D2			D3		
R1	R2	R3	R1	R2	R3	R1	R2	R3

	R1	R2	R3	R1	R2	R3	R1	R2	R3
S1									
S2									
S3									

S1 12″ beach ball D1 9′ R1 3′ arc
S2 8″ beach ball D2 18′ R2 5′ arc
S3 4″ beach ball D3 24′ R3 7′ arc

Figure 8-10. Grid evaluation for throwing Specific Task Analysis.

Task:
Kicking

Activity:
"Board Drop - Kick"

Equipment:
3 rubber utility balls,4",
    8", and 12" diameters
3 beach balls, 4", 8", and
    12" diameters
wall target 15' wide and 20'
    high, divided into 5 tar-
    get sectors, top and bot-
    tom sectors 2 feet high,
    center sector 8 feet high,
    inner sectors above and
    below center sector both
    4 feet high

Child's Task:
To drop-kick 1 of 5 balls
at a wall target 7 yards away.

The child should be able to
do this for:

1. Increasingly smaller sized balls.
2. Increasingly heavier balls.
3. Increasing accuracy.

Factors Influencing Student Performance			
	Size	Weight	Accuracy
Simple to **C**omplex (Levels)	S1 12" ball	W1 beach ball	A1 3 point rows
	S2 8" ball		A2 2 point rows
	S3 4" ball	W2 rubber utility ball	A3 1 point rows

Figure 8-11. Specific Task Analysis for kicking.

Assessment						
	A1		A2		A3	
	W1	W2	W1	W2	W1	W2
S1						
S2						
S3						

S1	12" ball	A1	3 point rows	W1	beach ball
S2	8" ball	A2	2 point rows	W2	rubber utility ball
S3	4" ball	A3	1 point rows		

Figure 8-12. Grid evaluation for kicking Specific Task Analysis.

Task:
Catching

Activity:
"Net-Catch"

Equipment:
8' x 10' decorative net
    attached to a 8' x
    1' dowel rod and
    suspended from a
    wall
2 standards
3 foam balls 12", 8", 4"
    diameters
tape lines 2 yards, 4 yards,
    and 6 yards from the
    front of the catching
    net

Child's Task:
To catch balls rolled down
an inclined net.

The child should be able to
do this for:

1. Increasingly smaller balls.
2. Increasingly faster moving balls.
3. Situations in which he must
   make increasingly greater locomotor spatial adjustments prior
   to catching.

Factors Influencing Student Performance			
	Ball Size	Inclination of the Net	Spatial Adjustment
Levels Simple to Complex	*S1* 12" ball	*I1* 60 degrees	*A1* 2 yds. in front
	S2 8" ball		*A2* 4 yds. in front
	S3 4" ball	*I2* 45 degrees	*A3* 6 yds. in front

Figure 8-13. Specific Task Analysis for catching.

Assessment						
	A1		*A2*		*A3*	
	I1	*I2*	*I1*	*I2*	*I1*	*I2*
S1						
S2						
S3						

S1 12" ball   *I1* 60 degrees   *A1* 2 yds. in front
S2   8" ball   *I2* 45 degrees   *A2* 4 yds. in front
S3   4" ball   *A3* 6 yds. in front

Figure 8-14. Grid evaluation for catching Specific Task Analysis.

REFERENCES

Adams. J. A., & Creamer, L. R. Anticipatory timing of continuous and discrete responses. *Journal of Experimental Psychology,* 1962, *63,* 84-90.

Cumbee, F. A. A factorial analysis of motor coordination. *Research Quarterly,* 1954, *25,* 412-420.

Fleishman, E. A. Dimensional analysis of movement reactions. *Journal of Experimental Psychology,* 1958, *55,* 438-453.

Gallahue, D. L. The relationship between perceptual and motor abilities. *Research Quarterly,* 1968, *39,* 948-952.

Herkowitz, J. The Moving Embedded Figures Test. *Research Quarterly,* 1973, *43,* 479-488.

Jackson, A. S. Factor analysis of selected muscular strength and motor performance tests. *Research Quarterly,* 1971, *42,* 164-172.

McCloy, C. H. A factor analysis of tests of endurance. *Research Quarterly,* 1956, *27,* 213-216.

Rarick, G. L. An analysis of speed factors in simple athletic activities. *Research Quarterly,* 1937, *8,* 89-105.

Rarick, G. L., & Dobbins, D. A. Basic components in the motor performance of children six to nine years of age. *Medicine and Science in Sports,* 1975, *7,* 105-110.

Ridenour, M. V. The influence of object size, speed, and direction on the perception of moving objects. *Research Quarterly,* 1974, *45,* 293-301.

Williams, H. G. *The effects of systematic variation of speed and direction of object flight and of skill and age upon visuo-perceptual judgements of moving objects in three-dimensional space.* Unpublished doctoral dissertation, University of Wisconsin at Madison, 1968.

9

Assessing the Motor Development of Children: Presentation and Critique of Tests

JACQUELINE HERKOWITZ

The quest to develop meaningful evaluative tools capable of monitoring the development of infants and children has long engaged educators and developmental psychologists. Indeed, evaluative tools have both helped researchers and provided starting places from which programs of educational experience were carried forward or constructed. Our purpose here is to examine six such tools. The first four, the Denver Developmental Screening Test, the Lincoln-Oseretsky Motor Development Scale, The Bayley Scales of Infant Development, and the Gesell Developmental Schedules traditionally have been used to evaluate developmental status, which includes motor components. The remaining two, the Ohio State University Scale of Intra-Gross Motor Assessment and the DeOreo Fundamental Motor Skills Inventory are two new, uniquely promising approaches to assessing the motor development of children.

Standardized Motor Development Tests

The Denver Developmental Screening Test, the Lincoln-Oseretsky Motor Development Scale, the Bayley Scales of Infant Development, and the Gesell Developmental Schedules have all enjoyed reasonable standardization. Each deserves to be critiqued and compared to the others.

Denver Developmental Screening Test (DDST)

The DDST (Buros, 1971; Frankenburg & Dodds, 1967; Frankenburg, Dodds, & Fandal, 1970) was designed to provide a simple, inexpensive, and fast means of diagnosing delayed development in children, birth through 6 years, which could be employed by a relatively untrained examiner. Other tests used to diagnose delayed development such as the Stanford-Binet, Revised Yale Development Schedule, Cattell Infant Intelligence Scale, and Bayley Scales of Infant Development did not have these advantages.

The DDST contains 105 items, but children tested are infrequently administered more than 20. The test is administered individually, and evaluates four sectors of the child's functioning.

1. *Gross Motor* evaluates the child's ability to
   sit, walk, broad jump, pedal a tricycle, throw
   a ball overhand, catch a bounced ball, hop
   on one foot, and balance on one foot.
2. *Fine Motor-Adaptive* evaluates the child's
   ability to stack cubes, reach for objects, and
   draw a man.
3. *Language* evaluates the child's ability to
   respond to a bell, imitate speech sounds
   and recognize colors.
4. *Personal-Social* evaluates the child's ability
   to dress with supervision and smile responsively.

On the DDST record form, each test item in the four sectors is designated by a bar, which indicates the ages at which 25, 50, 75, and 90 percent of the standardization population can perform the particular test item (see Figure 9-1). A child is tested on items in each of the four sectors which fall just before, on, or just after his age line. Testing is terminated when a child has three failures in the sector being tested, and several passes to the left of any failure. After testing, the results of a child's performance in each sector are categorized as normal, abnormal, or questionable. A child's performance in any sector is considered normal if he

passes at least one item which is intersected by his age line and
if he has no delays on any items in that sector (that is, no failures
to perform any item passed by more than 90 percent of children
his age). A child's performance in a sector is considered abnormal
if he has two or more delays in that sector. It is considered questionable if he is delayed in just one item in each sector.

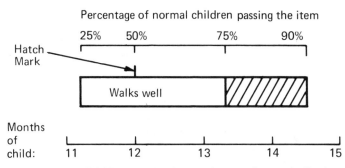

Figure 9-1. The DDST bar, indicating at what age the standardization
population performed the specific test item (here, walking.)

The standardization sample of 1036 children between the ages
of 2 weeks and 6.4 years, on which the original normative data
were collected, has been criticized as unrepresentative (Buros,
1971). It contained a significantly higher proportion of white
children and children whose fathers were in professional, mana-
gerial, and sales occupations than the census distribution would
warrant (Frankenburg, Dodds, & Fandal, 1970).

It also seems the DDST yields little more reliable information
than an interview with the mother would reveal (Buros, 1971;
Frankenburg, Camp, Van Natta, Demersseman, & Voorhees,
1971; Frankenburg, Dodds, & Fandal, 1970; Frankenburg,
Goldstein, & Camp, 1971). The test-retest reliabilities and interexaminer reliabilities reported in the accompanying manual were
based on extremely small samples of children (20 and 12, respec-

tively) representing a wide age range (2 months to 5½ years). Test-retest item agreement was 95.8 percent and the agreement for two examiners was reported as 90 percent (Frankenburg, Camp, Van Natta, Demersseman, & Voorhees, 1971). In this study, mental ages were calculated for 13 age groups between 1.5 and 49 months, using the 50 percent pass method for each of the four sectors. Coefficients ranged between 0.66 and 0.93. Test-retest reliabilities and interexaminer reliabilities proved generally poor when 1- and 2-year-olds were tested, but reached a more acceptable level in the testing of 3- and 4-year-olds. Interesting, however, of the 28 items with the highest tester-observer and test-retest reliabilities, 17 could be passed by report of the mother— yet only 5 of the 23 items with low tester-observer and test-retest reliabilities could be reported this way. The majority of the items on the DDST based on actual observations of the child's behavior were, at best, only moderately reliable.

Validity studies have been completed examining how the DDST agreed with other criterion tests in diagnosing developmental delays. The results of these analyses show a marked underselection by the DDST of under-30-month-old children who had received delayed development scores on the Bayley Scales of Infant Development and the Cattell Infant Intelligence Scale (Buros, 1971; Frankenburg, Camp, & Van Natta, 1971). Children over 30 months who were classified as abnormal on the Revised Yale Developmental Schedules and the Stanford-Binet were generally correctly identified on the DDST (Buros, 1971; Frankenburg, Camp, & Van Natta, 1971).

So—although easy to administer, and capable of being used by relatively untrained testers the DDST is not so reliable or valid as its authors had hoped. Its use for children under 30 months old should be discouraged because of questionable reliability at that age, and its inability to identify a high proportion of children identified as delayed by technically superior (although more lengthy) tests such as the Bayley and Cattell. It appears to be a fairly satisfactory screening tool for diagnosing delayed development in 4-year-olds.

Its usefulness as a motor development test is questionable in many ways. Gross motor and fine motor-adaptive items are assessed on a pass-fail basis. Developmental facets of each item, interesting to the educator, are often overlooked. For example, on the item, *throwing ball overhand,* the spinal rotation, arm-leg opposition, and sequential movement of body parts are of minimal significance. In the item, *catches bounced ball 2 or 3 times,* tracking ability and the efficiency of catching techniques demonstrated are not considered. Even after the *gross motor* and *fine motor-adaptive* items are evaluated, the test provides little definitive information to help direct those interested in remedying the problems of developmentally delayed youngsters.

Lincoln-Oseretsky Motor Development Scale

Five versions of the Oseretsky tests have been developed. The first version was published in 1923, in Russian, and the second was the 1945 Portuguese adaptation by DaCosta (Buros, 1959, 1974). The third version was an English translation of the Portuguese adaptation, by Fosa, which was published in 1946 (DaCosta, 1946*a-d*). Sloan provided the fourth version in 1948, popularly named the Lincoln-Oseretsky Motor Development Scale (Sloan, 1955). This test was based on the Fosa translation. The last version, by Bailer, Doll, and Winsberg (1973), was named the Modified Lincoln-Oseretsky Motor Development Scale.

The test is designed to provide a means by which relatively untrained examiners can assess the motor development status of children 5 through 15 years old. The most popular version, the Sloan version of 1955, contains 36 items, arranged in order of difficulty.

About two-thirds of the items consist of hand and arm movements—measuring speed, dexterity, coordination, and rhythm. The remainder are gross motor items: seven involving balance, and four testing jumping. The battery appears more heavily weighted toward manual coordination than this count would indicate, since a number of the manual items are scored for both the left and right hands. The question of what is actually being measured here has not been answered. Oseretsky (Sloan, 1955) claimed that his scale measured static coordination, dynamic coordination, and general speed of movement and asynkinesia; but no statistical support for his analysis was ever published. In factor analysis of Lincoln-Oseretsky scores on 211 boys 7½ to 11½ years of age, Thams (1955) found only one common factor accounting for about 20 percent of the variance. Age correlated with this factor 0.70, and Thams concluded that the factor was one of *motor development*. In a study on boys in grades 4-6, Carey (1954) obtained a correlation of 0.68 with grade and 0.37 with age. With three tests of gross motor ability, he obtained correlations of 0.32, 0.25, and 0.37. Low positive correlations were also obtained for height, weight, and IQ.

The similarity of scores for boys and for girls reported by Sloan (1955) and the low correlations with gross motor tests indicate that the Lincoln-Oseretsky scale does not measure strength or power. It can be considered a scale of motor development, since all the items sample a variety of motor performances and the scores improve with age.

Items are scored on a 0-to-3-point scale. A child's total score consists of all item points earned, added together. This scoring procedure is questionable. Although the maximum possible score on each test is 3 points, the only alternative score on 14 items is 0. Six items are scored 3-2-0, and the remaining 16, 3-2-1-0. There seems no logical reason for this variation, and it may create an unexpected weighting of some items in the total. Those who use the test should be aware of this possibility. The more recent Modified Lincoln-Oseretsky Motor Development Scale has only 26 of the original 36 items, with scoring criteria for 10 items changed to provide separate standards for each of seven age levels (Bailer, Doll, & Winsberg, 1973).

Sloan (1955) collected standardization data on 749 children, which he reported in his test manual. His findings included an analysis of each item retained from the original scale, the percentage of children passing each item at each age level, correlations of each item score with age (eta.), and tentative percentile norms for the sexes—separately and combined. He also noted odd-even reliabilities for boys and girls. The items in the scale were selected on the basis of their ability to discriminate between children of different ages. High internal consistency measures and odd-even reliability were reported by Sloan (1955). In addition, he calculated a mean test-retest reliability of 0.86.

Bailer, Doll, & Winsberg (1973) have shown that the Modified Lincoln-Oseretsky Motor Development Scale had split-half reliability coefficients between 0.69 and 0.89 for 5- through 11-year-old children.

The Lincoln-Oseretsky and the Modified Lincoln-Oseretsky scales should be considered valuable tools for studying certain aspects of motor development of school-age children. The fact that catching, striking, running, throwing, and kicking content are not included, however, may limit the tests' usefulness for some educators.

Bayley Scales of Infant Development (BSID)

The BSID (Bayley, 1969; Buros, 1971) is an individually administered test designed to assess the status of children 2 months to 2½ years of age. The BSID has been used in the recognition and diagnosis of sensory and neurological defects, and emotional disturbances.

The BSID consists of three parts: the *Mental Scale,* the *Motor Scale,* and the *Infant Behavior Record.* The Mental Scale is made up of 163 items which measure responses to visual and auditory stimuli, manipulation of and play with objects, and responses involving social interaction such as socialization and imitation. It also has items which measure discrimination of shapes, simple problem solving, and more abstract abilities such as naming objects, understanding prepositions, and the concept of the number one. The Motor Scale consists of 81 items which measure progressions of gross motor abilities such as sitting, standing, walking, and stair climbing; as well as abilities involving finer motor coordination, such as grasping objects of various sizes. The Infant Behavior Record is a rating scale which measures various aspects of personality, emotional and social behaviors, activity level, responses to objects, areas of interest, attention span, and persistence.

Unlike the Lincoln-Oseretsky or DDST tests, the BSID materials are very expensive. Several items on the Motor Scale require the construction of apparatus (such as a specially constructed staircase and a walking board).

The greatest advantage of the BSID over other tests of development lies in its excellent standardization. The standardization sample was large and representative of the United States population in terms of major geographical areas, urban-rural areas, sex, race, and education of the head of the household (Bayley, 1969; Buros, 1971). Its test manual is specific, clear, and logical.

On the other hand, the BSID is difficult to learn to administer because of the overwhelming amount of information one must keep in mind while giving it. Not only do so many items in the scales make administration difficult, but also the variety of factors to remember in the instructions may make the scale seem formidable to an inexperienced tester. The items are arranged on the scales in order of age difficulty. In general, a child is tested over items 1 month earlier than his chronological age and upward. The experimenter's task is to locate the most difficult items the child can pass.

The test (Motor and Mental Scales) usually takes about 45 minutes, although about 10 percent of cases require 75 minutes or more. Scoring of the BSID is straightforward. Items on the Motor and Mental Scales are given a credit of 1 if a child can pass them. These raw scores can easily be converted into index scores which allow comparisons of a child's performance on the Mental Scale and Motor Scale with those of children of the same age who were members of the standardization sample. These indices are respectively termed the *Mental Development Index* and the *Psychomotor Development Index*. A series of scales are used for rating significant behaviors demonstrated on the Infant Behavior Record. The record requires the examiner to make a combination of specific observations and qualitative judgements and is often used when clinical decisions need to be made, to supplement the results of the Motor and Mental Scales.

The Mental Scale scores on the BSID correlate substantially with those on the Stanford-Binet (Bayley, 1969). No published predictive validity information is available on the Mental Scale, and no validity data are available on the Motor Scale.

The split-half reliability of the Mental and Motor Scales, as determined for 14 age groups, ranged from 0.68 to 0.93 (Bayley, 1969). BSID items which have the highest tester-observer and test-retest reliability are those (1) having to do with eye-hand coordination directed toward a test object, (2) treating sustained attention toward a test object, and (3) involving object constancy and vocabulary items. Low test-retest and tester-observer reliability was found on motor scale items that required an examiner's assistance (Bayley, 1969; Buros, 1971).

Although this test has been used for decades, its usefulness for those predominantly interested in the motor development of children is questionable. Certainly it is designed to assess only very young children. As noted above, its weakest test-retest reliability was found on motor scale items requiring an examiner's assistance. Probably those who included the items on the test and those who administer them do not perceive fully the enormous influence of equipment and directions on the performance of motor skills early in life. Until this weakness is corrected, the reliability of this test will always be suspect. To compound the problem, there is no published validity data on the Motor Scale.

Gesell Developmental Schedules (GDS)

The GDS (Buros, 1949, 1953, 1965; Gesell & Amatruda, 1949) have been used predominantly in following up on infants with complications at birth or as predictors of intellectual development in the preschool and early school years. The GDS are individually administered and appropriate for use with children 4 weeks to 6 years of age.

The developmental schedules are presented as lists of behavior items ordered according to developmental maturity, and against which a child's behavior is compared. There are four fields of normative behavior to which children to be assessed are compared: *Motor, Adaptive, Language,* and *Personal-Social.* Each of the ten standard forms presents three adjacent ages in vertical alignment, subdivided into the four fundamental behavior categories. This arrangement permits cross-comparison for separate fields of behavior. One applies the schedules simply by determining how well a child's behavior fits one age-level constellation of behavior rather than another; he *compares* the child to the schedules. Single items do not have age values—are not weighted, added, or subtracted. The aggregate picture is sought. If a child's maturity levels on examination are shown to be Motor, 36 months; Adaptive, 42 months; Language, 30 months; and Personal-Social, 30-36 months, then the maturity levels are represented this way—not in a composite manner or by one score.

There is a standard order for administering the behavior test situations. The situations sequences are adapted to maturity differences characteristic of five broad age periods: supine, sitting, locomotor, prekindergarten, and kindergarten. In addition, a special set of five analytical forms are available which list increasing, decreasing, and focal behavior items for fifteen age levels, from 4 through 56 weeks. These deal with postural, prehensory, perceptual, adaptive, and language-social behavior.

Information on standardization procedures and the norms and instructions for administering and scoring the GDS are scattered in three different volumes. One of these is out of print (Gesell & Amatruda, 1947; Gesell & Thompson, 1938; Gesell *et al.,* 1940). Possibly the very high cost of the test materials—which is considerably over $100.00 now—would be lower if the administration, scoring, and other standardization materials were consolidated in one concise volume. Also, the standardization data were collected three decades ago, so a restandardization on a large sample of United States infants would help today. Over the past three decades, there may well have been a change in the typical pattern of infant behavior, possibly resulting from better nutritional status, pediatric care, and changed child rearing practices (Buros, 1965).

A number of validity studies have been completed on the GDS. Taken together, they indicate that the Gesell schedules have high concurrent validity and low predictive validity. Knobloch and Pasamanick (1960) reported a high correlation between the Gesell and the Stanford-Binet ($r = 0.97$, $n = 195$) for 3-year-old children. This is not surprising, however, since a number of items in the GDS at the 3-year-old level were taken directly from the Binet test. Gardener and Swiger (1958) found in a study of 128 infants, age 4 to 92 days, a moderately high negative correlation (-0.64) between Developmental Quotients and Chronological Age, indicating that the GDS are inadequate discriminators during the early weeks of infancy. Follow-up studies of infants tested when younger than 8 months have shown the GDS to have little predictive value. Escalona and Moriarty (1961) found no relationship between GDS scores and normal infants tested between 3 weeks and 33 weeks and retested between 6 and 9 years. Share, Webb, and Koch (1961) found that the Developmental Quotients for Mongoloids tested at median age of 7.5 months are not good predictors of later Developmental Quotients. In contrast, however, the Developmental Quotients of the same 16 Mongoloids tested at median age 17.0 months and median age 29.5 months yielded a correlation of 0.86. Knobloch and Pasamanick (1960) report a correlation of 0.51 between GDS scores of 40-week-old infants and their 3-year GDS scores (0.74 for 48 abnormal infants and 0.43 for 147 normal infants). Correlations between 40-week GDS scores and 3-year Binet scores are in the same range ($r = 0.48$, $n = 195$). The same investigators report a correlation of 0.50 between 40-week GDS scores and 7-year intelligence test scores. Simon and Bass (1956) obtained essentially similar results by classifying infants' Gesell scores into three categories (dull, average, above average). It appears difficult to predict later intellectual status from early GDS performance.

Very little reliability data are available on the GDS. Knoblock and Pasamanick (1960) report the only reliability data found: correlations between the Developmental Quotients obtained by the examiner and several observers (all trained by the same examiner). Two sets of correlations were computed: one for clinical cases (one-third abnormal), the other for normal infants participating in a longitudinal follow-up study. The correlations reported varied from 0.90 to 0.99 on samples of 40-week-old infants with numbers ranging from 12 to 44. These tester-observer reliability coefficients were surprisingly high, considering the vagueness of the scoring methods. There is a need for both tester-observer and test-retest reliability studies at different age levels (Buros, 1949, 1953, 1965).

The GDS should not be considered an infant and preschool intelligence test, because predictions about future development, especially intellectual development, cannot be made from the schedules with any certainty. Evidence accumulated suggests that predictions are extremely hazardous, particularly in the very youngest age ranges. The questionable reliability also severely limits the schedules' usefulness, as does the need for an extensive revision drawn from a large and representative sample of present-day infants. This test, like the Bayley, is also limited by insensitivity to biomechanical and psychomotor learning factors that most certainly must have influenced the reliability of motor items.

Conclusions

The tests presented represent four traditional attempts to evaluate developmental status. All include motor components, and all have enjoyed considerable use. All are individually administered, but the Lincoln-Oseretsky, Modified Lincoln-Oseretsky, and DDST require considerably less administration time than the others. The BSID and GDS require extensive examiner training;

the DDST and the Lincoln-Oseretsky tests do not. Only the Lincoln-Oseretsky test, of the four, exclusively contains gross and fine motor content.

None of the tests lend themselves to use with a wide age range of children. The BSID is only useful with children under 2½ years of age, the GDS and DDST are useful only with children through 6 years of age, and the Lincoln-Oseretsky tests are good for children 5 through 15 years of age. Since the BSID is designed for very young children, it is not surprising to see postural control, locomotion, and prehensile activity emphasized. The lack of substantive attention to striking, catching, throwing, jumping, running, and kicking behaviors evidenced on the GDS, Lincoln-Oseretsky, and DDST, however, have probably limited their use by those predominantly interested in the movement behavior of normal children.

All four tests are structured around the concept of age-appropriate behavior. Items in the four tests were selected to identify which behaviors should be expected of children at different ages. This concept contrasts sharply with promising new assessment devices based on developmental biomechanical information which ask testers to place children along developmental continua in the fundamental motor categories of striking, throwing, jumping, climbing, catching, and running—without denoting such "age-appropriate" expectations (Loovis, 1975). This approach promises relief for the barraged teacher, and acknowledges openly the great variability in the time young children take to acquire efficient movement behavior.

Although these four tests are, for the most part, well standardized, it is not by accident that their fine and gross motor content is often their least reliable, least valid material. Those who originated these tests simply did not possess the biomechanic and motor learning specialists' sensitivity to the enormous influence of equipment and directions on the performance of what are predominantly phylogenetic activities early in life. Until the influence of (1) equipment, and (2) verbal, visual, and manual guidance on motor behavior of young children is investigated, the motor content in these tests will probably remain weak.

New Directions in Motor Development Assessment

Two more recently developed, although not well standardized, evaluative attempts seem particularly promising. These are the *Ohio State University Scale of Intra-Gross Motor Assessment* (Loovis, 1975) and the *DeOreo Fundamental Motor Skills Inventory* (DeOreo, 1976). The first test attempts to assess the child's efficiency of performance in 11 skill categories, while the second one seeks to judge the efficiency of motor skill performances and the products of those performances in 11 categories.

Ohio State University Scale of Intra-Gross Motor Assessment (OSU Sigma)

The OSU Sigma (Loovis, 1975) was designed to assess the efficiency and maturity of preschool through 14-year-old children's performance on 11 selected gross motor skills: walking, catching, ladder climbing, stair climbing, throwing, striking, skipping, running, hopping, jumping, and kicking. The performance of a child on any one of the 11 selected gross motor skills is assessed by comparing observations of the child's performance in a setting and with equipment noted in the test, with descriptions of behaviors ordered from less efficient and mature to more efficient and mature. Each skill on the OSU Sigma Test is presented on a single page. At the top, equipment for administering the item is noted and the necessary testing conditions are defined. Descriptions of performance are presented in each of four columns, labeled *Level I, Level II, Level III,* and *Level IV,* representing least to most efficient behavior. The gross motor skill of stair climbing is presented in Figure 9-2.

To date, no validity data and only limited reliability data exist for the OSU Sigma Test. A test-retest reliability study was reported by Loovis (1975). Thirteen judges viewed and rated the video-taped performance of 12 normal children, ages 2 through 14 years, on the OSU Sigma Test, on two occasions separated by a 1-week interval. Data were analyzed with Scott's Pi.

SKILL OF STAIR CLIMBING

TEST EQUIPMENT: Series of Stairs

LEVEL I	LEVEL II	LEVEL III	LEVEL IV
When positioned at the bottom of a series of steps,	When standing at the bottom of a series of steps,	Same	Same

Note: Examiner cannot serve as an aid in place of railing or wall . . . .

LEVEL I	LEVEL II	LEVEL III	LEVEL IV
The child demonstrates one of the following behaviors:	The child, with or without the aid of the railing or wall, walks up and down 5 steps and demonstrates the following behaviors in two out of three trials:	The child, with the aid of the railing or wall, walks up and down 5 steps and demonstrates the following behaviors in two out of three trials:	The child independently walks up and down 5 steps and demonstrates the following behaviors in two out of three trials:
a. creeps up 5 steps and slides down from step to step on the buttock	a. walks up using two-foot landing (mark-time pattern)	a. walks up using an alternate stepping pattern	a. walks up using an alternate stepping pattern
b. creeps up and down 5 steps	b. walks down either in the same manner or by sliding from step to step on the buttock	b. walks down in the same manner or by using a two-foot landing (mark-time pattern)	b. walks down using an alternate stepping pattern
c. walks up and back down while in a hands-feet position like animal walking			

Figure 9-2. The gross motor skill of stair climbing, as presented on the OSU Sigma Test.

Pi coefficients for interjudge and intrajudge test reliability for each of the 11 skills were classified into three groups. Walking, catching, ladder climbing, and stair climbing each had a median Pi reliability coefficient of 0.83 or higher. This group of skills was identified as having high reliability. The group with medium reliability coefficients (0.54 to 0.82) included throwing, striking, and skipping. The group with low reliability coefficients (0.53 or lower) included running, hopping, jumping, and kicking. In short, the high reliability group of walking, catching, ladder climbing, and stair climbing had reliability coefficients within the range of acceptability, but the others produced reliability coefficients lower than conventional standards. Percentage of agreement among judges on the first administration of the test indicated that walking, catching, ladder climbing, and stair climbing had 0.91 or higher agreement. Throwing, striking, and skipping had 0.75 agreement. All other items had between 0.50 and 0.67 agreement. It would seem that more careful delineation of directions and appropriate testing equipment might increase the interjudge and intrajudge reliability of the OSU Sigma Test. Equipment requirements and the directions the tester is to give to the child are not always clear in each of the items.

The OSU Sigma Test, although not well standardized, does seem a promising approach to assessment for those interested in motor development. The validity of the stage concept of development of a gross motor skill on which the test is based was supported by the research of Roberton (1976). She noted that stage theory in motor development predicts that human movement changes over time in immutable sequential stages, and she supported this belief with biomechanical studies of the overhand throwing behavior of children. In addition, it is possible that future use of the multivariate procedures of seriation and one-dimensional multidimensional scaling [Johnson, 1968; Korell & Safrit, 1977; Kruskal, 1964 (a and b)] may provide a statistical means of validating the OSU Sigma Test. Future reliability studies based on the coefficient *kappa* (Swaninathan, Hambleton, & Algina, 1974) may provide even more meaningful insights into the agreement between the decisions made in repeated test administrations. This statistic is appropriate for use when scores are not necessarily expected to vary widely and when one is concerned with whether or not subjects are being classified in the same way from one time to another, as is the case here.

An additional strength of the OSU Sigma Test is that it is not administered in contrived laboratory settings or strange environments. This feature may contribute to its validity and ease of administration. It may also encourage its use in school settings where complex, time-consuming, and contrived instruments are difficult to use or inappropriate. The data derived from the OSU Sigma Test should also have direct application in evaluation and planning aspects of school curriculum.

DeOreo Fundamental Motor Skills Inventory (DFMSI)

Recently DeOreo (1976) devised a developmental assessment instrument called the DFMSI for use with preschool children. The DFMSI examines performance in 11 categories: striking, balancing, skipping, jumping, galloping, hopping, catching, running, climbing, throwing, and kicking. Items to be assessed under each gross motor category are divided into *product components,* such as "Can the child run 35 yards in less than 10 seconds?" and *process components,* such as "While running does the child keep his body erect or inclined backwards?" All the process and product components to be assessed under each gross motor category are noted on a single sheet with space allocated to the right for the examiner to check "Yes," "Sometimes," or "No," in response to each component (see Figure 9-3).

The test also provides a scoring and interpretation sheet for each of the 11 gross motor categories. This sheet assigns point values to items accomplished normally by 3-, 4-, and 5-year-olds (see Figure 9-4). When a child's performance is assessed, for every "Yes" answer on the inventory sheet he or she is assigned appropriate point values. The total score is then compared to

RUNNING

Product Components:

1. Can the child run 35 yards in less than 10 seconds?
2. Can the child run 35 yards in less than 20 seconds?
3. Can the child run 35 yards in less than 30 seconds?

Process Components:

4. While running does the child:
   a. experience difficulty in controlling starts, stops, and sudden turns?
   b. control starting, stopping, and sudden turns most of the time?
   c. control starting, stopping, and sudden turns with ease?

5. Does the child run:
   a. with flat foot pattern?
   b. using the balls of his feet to push in forward direction?
   c. receiving his weight on the whole foot?
   d. receiving his weight on the ball of his foot?
   e. with his toes pointed outward?
   f. with his toes pointed forward in the direction of movement?

6. While running are the arms of the child:
   a. bent and moving in a back and forth, sideways direction across body?
   b. bent, swinging freely, and moving in opposition?

7. While running does the child keep his body:
   a. erect or inclined backward?
   b. inclined slightly forward?

(Columns: Yes / Sometimes / No)

Figure 9-3. The DFMSI examination sheet for the gross motor skill of running.

RUNNING
Points for Yes Answers Only
(age in years)

	3	4	5
1.			3
2.		2	
3.	1		
4.a.	1		
b.		2	
c.			3
5.a.	1		
b.		2	
c.	1		
d.			3
e.	1		
f.		2	
6.a.		2	
b.			3
7.a.	1		
b.			3

The items on the inventory are represented at the right, and the age at which each specific item should be mastered by the pre-school child is designated.

Point values have been assigned to the items with 1 point scored for those items ordinarily performed by 3-year-olds, 2 points for items ordinarily performed by 4-year-olds and 3 points for items ordinarily performed by 5-year-olds.

The 3-year-old child should be able to perform items: 3, 4a, 5a, 5c, 5e, 6a, and 7a. The 4-year-old child should be able to master items: 2, 4b, 5b, 5f, and 6a. The 5-year-olds should be able to perform items 1, 4c, 5d, 6b, and 7b.

For each of the "yes" answers on the inventory sheet, assign the appropriate point value and total all points. Find the score on the following scale.

SCORE	AGE OF CHILD		
	36-47 months	48-59 months	60-71 months
1-5	Below average	Remedial	Remedial
6-7	Average	Poor	Remedial
8-9	Above average	Below average	Remedial
10-11	Good	Average	Poor
12-14	Excellent	Above average	Below average
15-16	Outstanding	Good	Average

Children that are designated as below average may or may not need motor training, as this score may merely reflect the variability in performance that is typical of young children. However, children designated as poor and remedial are children in need of motor training and should be given special attention and guidance in specific motor activities designed to bring their motor performance into the normal range.

Figure 9-4. The DEMSI scoring and interpretation sheet for running.

age level, and performance is labeled *poor, remedial, below average, average, above average, good, excellent,* or *outstanding.*

DeOreo's (1976) determinations about appropriate behaviors associated with 3-, 4-, and 5-year-olds were derived from reading literature regarding performance standards and developmental biomechanics for preschool children. To date, no standardization data are available on the inventory. Freedman (1976) has administered the throwing item from the DFMSI to 28 graduate students, and calculated interrater reliability in terms of percent agreement of raters. The raters rated 5 children throwing 10 trials each of a forceful overhand throw. Rater agreement for the various sections of the item was calculated. However, overall agreement was 0.47. This was considered unacceptably low. It would seem that with time, careful delineation of equipment and validity data will be presented. Perhaps,too, the relationship between process and product components of performance will be clarified as the test undergoes standardization.

Conclusions

Both the DFMSI and the OSU Sigma Test offer strong process-oriented approaches to motor development assessment. The OSU Sigma Test emphasizes the need to recognize the stages of efficient and mature motor skill acquisition, and acknowledges the great variability demonstrated by young children. The DFMSI attempts to consider both process and product components,and provides a means by which the age-appropriateness of performance can be assessed. Both assessment techniques seem to be easily usable in school settings by relatively untrained examiners. Once both evaluative devices have undergone further development and rigorous standardization, proving themselves reliable and valid, they should become valuable tools for those interested in the assessment of motor development.

REFERENCES

Bailer, I., Doll, L., & Winsberg, B. G. *Modified Lincoln-Oseretsky Motor Development Scale.* New York: New York State Department of Mental Hygiene, 1973.

Bayley, N. *Manual for the Bayley Scales of Infant Development.* New York: The Psychological Corporation, 1969.

Buros, O. K., ed. *The third mental measurements yearbook.* Highland Park, N. J.: Gryphon, 1949, entry 276.

Buros, O. K., ed. *The fourth mental measurements yearbook.* Highland Park, N. J.: Gryphon, 1953, entry 341.

Buros, O. K., ed. *The fifth mental measurements yearbook.* Highland Park, N. J.: Gryphon, 1959, entry 767.

Buros, O. K., ed. *The sixth mental measurements yearbook.* Highland Park, N. J.: Gryphon, 1965, entry 522.

Buros. O. K., ed. *The seventh mental measurements yearbook.* Highland Park, N. J.: Gryphon, 1971, entry 405.

Buros, O. K., ed. *Tests in Print II.* Highland Park, N. J.: Gryphon, 1974, entry 1895.

Carey, R. A. A comparison of the Lincoln Revision of the Oseretsky Test of Motor Proficiency with selected motor ability tests on boys at the elementary level. Unpublished doctoral dissertation, Indiana University, 1954.

DaCosta, M. I. The Oseretsky tests: Method, value, and results (Portuguese adaptation). Elizabeth Joan Fosa, tr., *Training School Bulletin,* 1946 (*a*), *43,* 1-13.

DaCosta, M. I. The Oseretsky tests, Part II. Elizabeth Joan Fosa, tr., *Training School Bulletin,* 1946 (*b*), *43,* 27-38.

DaCosta, M. I. The Oseretsky tests, Part III. Elizabeth Joan Fosa, tr., *Training School Bulletin,* 1946 (*c*), *43,* 50-59.

DaCosta, M. I. The Oseretsky tests, Part IV. Elizabeth Joan Fosa, tr., *Training School Bulletin,* 1946 (*d*), *43,* 62-74.

DeOreo, K. L. Unpublished current work on the assessment of the development of gross motor skills, Kent State University, 1976.

Escalona, S. K., & Moriarty, A. Prediction of school-age intelligence from infant tests. *Child Development,* 1961, *32,* 597-605.

Frankenburg, W. K., Camp, B. W., & Van Natta, P. A. Validity of the Denver Developmental Screening Test. *Child Development,* 1971, *42,* 475-485.

Frankenburg, W. K., Camp, B. W., Van Natta, P. A., Demmersseman, J. A., & Voorhees, S. F. Reliability and stability of the Denver Developmental Screening Tests. *Child Development,* 1971, *42,* 1315-1325.

Frankenburg, W. K., & Dodds, J. B. The Denver Developmental Screening Test. *Journal of Pediatrics,* 1967, *71,* 181-191.

Frankenburg, W. K., Dodds, J. B., & Fandal, A. W. *Denver Developmental Screening Test.* Boulder, Col.: University of Colorado Medical Center, 1970.

Frankenburg, W., Goldstein, A. D., & Camp, B. W. The revised Denver Developmental Screening Test: Its accuracy as a screening instrument. *Journal of Pediatrics,* 1971, *79,* 988-995.

Freedman, M. S. Assessing inter-rater reliability for the throwing item in the *DeOreo Fundamental Motor Skills Inventory.* Unpublished paper, Ohio State University, 1976.

Gardener, D. B., & Swiger, M. K. Developmental status of two groups of infants released for adoption. *Child Development,* 1958, *29,* 521-530.

Gesell, A., & Amatruda, C. S. *Developmental Diagnosis.* New York: Harper & Row, 1947.

Gesell, A., & Amatruda, C. S. *Gesell Developmental Schedules.* New York: Psychological Company, 1949.

Gesell, A., & Thompson, H. *The Psychology of Early Growth.* New York: MacMillan, 1938.

Gesell, A., *et al. The First Five Years of Life.* New York: Harper & Row, 1940.

Johnson, L. Jr. Item seriation as an aid for elementary scale and cluster analysis. *Museum of Natural History,* University of Oregon Bulletin, 1968, 15.

Knoblock, H., & Pasamanick, B. An evaluation of the consistency and pre-dictive value of the 40-week Gesell Developmental Schedule. In Shagass, C., & Pasamanick, B., eds. *Child Development and Child Psychiatry.* Washington, D. C.: American Psychiatric Associates, 1960.

Korell, D. M., & Safrit, M. J. A comparison of seriation and multidimen-sional scaling: Two techniques for validating construction in physical education. *Research Quarterly,* in press.

Kruskal, J. B. Multidimensional scaling by optimizing goodness of fit to a nonmetric hypothesis, I. *Psychometrika,* 1964 (*a*), *29,* 1-27.

Kruskal, J. B. Multidimensional scaling by optimizing goodness of fit to a nonmetric hypothesis, II. *Psychometrika,* 1964 (*b*), *29,* 115-129.

Loovis, E. M. Model for individualizing physical education experiences for the preschool moderately retarded child. (Doctoral dissertation, The Ohio State University, 1975). *Dissertation Abstracts International,* 1976, *36* 5126A (University Microfilms No. 76-3485).

Roberton, M. A. Stability of stage categorizations across trials: Implications for the "stage theory" of overarm throw development (Doctoral dissertation, University of Wisconsin at Madison, 1975). *Dissertation Abstracts International,* 1976, *36,* 5291A (University Microfilms No. 75-20, 792).

Share, J., Webb, A., & Koch, R. A preliminary investigation of the early developmental status of Mongoloid infants. *American Journal of Mental Deficiency,* 1961, *66,* 238-241.

Simon, A. J., & Bass, L. G. Toward a validation of infant testing. *American Journal of Orthopsychiatry,* 1956, *26,* 340-350.

Sloan, W. The Lincoln-Oseretsky Motor Development Scale. *Genetic Psychology Monographs,* 1955, *51,* 183-252.

Swaninathan, H., Hambleton, R. K., & Algina, J. Reliability of criterion-referenced tests: A decision-theoretic formulation. *Journal of Educational Measurement,* 1974, *11,* 263-266.

Thams, P. F. A factor analysis of the Lincoln-Oseretsky Motor Development Scale. Unpublished doctoral dissertation, University of Michigan, 1955.

Appendices

A

Locating and Retrieving
Literature in Motor Development

MARCELLA V. RIDENOUR

The location and retrieval of literature is a prerequisite to excellence in teaching and research in motor development and motor learning. This appendix has two sections, one describing general procedures for all searches, and one describing specific indices. A complete search will involve the following indices:

> *Index to Scientific Reviews*
> *Psychological Abstracts*
> *Child Development Abstracts and Bibliography*
> *Dissertation Abstracts International*
> *Resources in Education*
> *Social Sciences Citation Index*
> *Index Medicus*
> *Health, Physical Education, and Recreation Microcard
>   Bulletin*
> *Completed Research in Health, Physical Education, and
>   Recreation*
> *Abstracts of Research Papers*

The Procedure

The procedure for initiating a literature search involves determining the scope and limitations of the topic and identifying key words. The searcher should review textbooks relating to the topic and identify basic books and specialists in the area. If he or she writes to these specialists, he may be rewarded with excellent bibliographies and unpublished reports and chapters.

The next procedure in the search is locating relevant review articles in the *Index to Scientific Reviews*. After carefully examining these articles, he can then turn to *Psychological Abstracts* and the *Child Development Index* as excellent sources for identifying completed research in motor learning and motor development and to *Dissertation Abstracts International* for relevant doctoral dissertations. If the researcher does locate a relevant dissertation, it may take him 3 to 5 weeks to obtain a complete copy of it.

After determining both basic and classical references and specialists identified with his or her selected topic, the scholar might then look at the *Social Sciences Citation Index* to check the completeness of his literature review. The search is complete only when all sources and references merely duplicate prior references. *Index Medicus* is an excellent source for articles and references not described in other sources, although searching there is a very long, time-consuming process. Most major medical school libraries have on-line computer searches of *Index Medicus* at a very reasonable cost.

Since *Dissertation Abstracts* omits theses leading to a Master's degree and many doctoral dissertations, the researcher will also want to look at the *Health, Physical Education and Recreation Microcard Bulletin,* and *Completed Research in Health, Physical Education and Recreation* to locate theses and dissertations completed in physical education.

Also, many unpublished papers are presented at the National Convention of the American Alliance for Health, Physical Education and Recreation, and published in the *Abstracts of Research Papers.*

A scholarly literature search assumes the review and critique of original references. A literature review based primarily on indirect and incomplete references such as textbooks, review articles, and abstracts tends to involve frequent inaccuracies or misrepresentations. A researcher and/or teacher must be able to communicate the *complete* design and experimental results to other researchers and inquisite students, and so he should fall back on a secondary source only when either the primary source is not available or there is no translation from a foreign language.

Remember, too, that indices generally take 2 to 6 months to index and abstract a periodical after it is published, so a complete literature search involves going through the yet-to-be-indexed periodicals of the past 6 months. A weekly periodical, *Current Contents in Social and Behavioral Sciences,* will assist with the search for current references by providing a copy of the table of contents for all periodicals published in *Social and Behavioral Sciences* during the past week. Addresses of the authors are also given for quick access to reprints, and the publisher offers a quick reprint service for a minimal charge. Most libraries subscribe to *Current Contents in the Social and Behavioral Sciences,* but the name and address of the publisher is Institute for Scientific Information, 325 Chestnut Street, Philadelphia, Pa. 19106.

Major Indices

The second part of this appendix, to which we now turn, involves the listing and description of major indices relevant to motor development and motor learning research.

Name:	**Index to Scientific Reviews (ISR)**
Address:	Institute for Scientific Information
	325 Chestnut Street
	Philadelphia, Pa. 19106

Published semiannually (cumulated annually)
Annual cost: $250.00
Available from 1974

The Index to Scientific Reviews (ISR) retrieves significant review articles published throughout the world on any subject in science. Each year ISR indexes over 20,000 review articles appearing in 2600 of the world's most important scientific journals. ISR also covers literature published in quarterly and annual "review" publications.

Four basic types of searches can be performed with the Index to Scientific Reviews. The most complete search would incorporate several of these.

Citation Searching (*Citation Index*)

Citation searching is best used when the searcher already knows an earlier key author, paper, book, or other relevant published material. He or she starts with a reference or author that is familiar, turns to the Citation Index section, and looks for that particular name. If starting with an author, when he locates the author's name, he then checks to see which of the possible cited references fits the particular subject matter in which he is interested. Under the year, journal, volume, and page number of this particular reference, he then looks to see which review author has currently cited this particular work. Having noted the bibliographical citations of the review authors who have cited the work with which he started, the searcher then turns to the Source Index section and obtains the complete bibliographical data for the desired review articles.

Subject Searching (*Permuterm Subject Index*)

Subject searching can help most when no earlier relevant papers or authors on a subject are known. This approach is particularly important for researchers entering a new field. In the Permuterm Subject Index each significant word, or, in some cases, word-phrase, is listed alphabetically as a main entry or primary term, and is also paired with all other significant words in a title (as secondary or co-terms) with which the primary term has co-occurred. Each such permuted word pair is linked to the name of a first author who has used the word pair in the title of a published review article covered in the Source Index. The Permuterm Subject Index serves as a natural language, terminologically current title-word index, and permits a rapid subject search of the review literature.

For example, selecting *motor* and *development* as the pair of terms with which to begin the search, the following entry is located in the Permuterm Subject Index of the ISR.

Under MOTOR   Development   Asanuma, H.

At this point the searcher notes the name of the author and looks it up in the Source Index section of the ISR to get a full description of the article.

Author Searching (*Source Index*)

The searcher can try author searching when he or she knows the name of an author of a review article, but nothing about which publication the review article appeared in, or when he knows a specific author periodically writes reviews in his field of interest. He simply looks up the author in the Source Index.

Organization Searching (*Source Index*)

Through organization searching, a researcher can identify quickly all the review articles from a given organization that have been published during the period indexed. Once he or she looks up the names of the published authors from the organization he can obtain full information on the review articles they have published from the Source Index.

Name: **Psychological Abstracts**
Address: American Psychological Association, Inc.
             1200 17th Street N. W.
             Washington, D. C. 20036

Published monthly
Annual cost: $190.00
Available from 1927

Psychological Abstracts covers over 850 journals, technical reports, monographs, and other scientific documents. It provides nonevaluative abstracts of world literature in psychology and related disciplines.

Monthly issues contain 17 major categories, some with subsections. Major categories include *perception and motor performance, developmental psychology, neurology, and physiology and educational psychology.* Under each classification heading, the abstracts are arranged alphabetically by first author. Abstracts that are relevant to a major category but not to any of the subsections are listed first; these are followed by abstracts relevant to both major category and subsections.

Psychological Abstracts includes an Author Index and a brief Subject Index which refer readers to the abstracts mentioned above. Entries in the Subject Index are derived from a 4,000 word Thesaurus of Psychological Index terms. Each entry also refers the reader to more specific concepts related to each term. For instance, a user interested in motor development would also be referred to psychomotor development and speech development, provided there are entries in those areas.

Name:	**Child Development Abstracts and Bibliography**
Address:	University of Chicago Press
	5801 Ellis Avenue
	Chicago, Ill. 60637

Published three times per year
Annual cost: $10.00
Available from 1927

Child Development Abstracts and Bibliography contains abstracts of articles in eight categories: *biology, including infancy; clinical medicine and public health; developmental and comparative psychology; experimental psychology, including learning phenomena; personality; sociology and social psychology; education, educational psychology, and counseling;* and *psychiatry, clinical psychology, and other clinical studies.*

The subject index is set up from a controlled vocabulary. Since *motor development* is a term, you would be referred to abstract numbers in this area. An author index provides abstract numbers as well.

Also included are book notices (abstracts), books received (which acknowledge items received by CDAB but not yet issued for review), and lists of (1) journals abstracted in the current issue, and (2) periodicals regularly searched.

Name:	**Dissertation Abstracts International**
	Section A. Humanities and Social Sciences
	Section B. Physical Sciences and Technology
Address:	University Microfilms, Xerox Company
	300 N. Zeeb Road
	Ann Arbor, Mich. 48106

Published monthly

Annual cost:	$175.00 for both sections ($110.00 microfiche)
	$105.00 separate ($67.50 microfiche)

Available from 1938

Beginning with volume 30; no. 1, the title *Dissertation Abstracts* was changed to *Dissertation Abstracts International.* It is a monthly compilation of doctoral dissertations submitted to Xerox University Microfilms by over 350 cooperating institutions in the United States and Canada.

Dissertation Abstracts International is divided into two sections: *Humanities (A)* and *Sciences (B).* Both are arranged by broad subject categories, and the dissertation author chooses the category which most nearly describes the general content of the dissertation. The main categories for Section A are: *communi-*

cations and the arts; education; language; literature, and linguistics; philosophy, religion and theology; and *social science.* For Section B the categories are *biological sciences; earth sciences, health and environmental sciences, physical sciences and psychology.*

The Table of Contents lists in alphabetical order the principal subject categories of the dissertations abstracted. A Keyword Title Index and an Author Index are included following the abstracts. The keyword index has the bibliographical entries classified and arranged alphabetically by important words contained in the title. The keywords are printed in boldface type and are followed by the titles in which they occur. In addition, the subject category chosen by the author, the author's name, and page reference are given after each title to facilitate location of the article. Similarly, the author index refers the reader to section and page number.

The keyword *motor* in the Section A title index provided the following reference:

MOTOR
A comparison of the differences in motor and cognitive development between educationally high risk children at the conclusion of Piaget's sensori-motor stage.
(Education, Special)
Schoonover, Robert Jay, p. 224A

For this particular search, one would want to consult Section B in the same manner.

Name:	**ERIC Resources in Education (RIE)**
	(Changed from *Research in Education* in January 1975)
Address:	Educational Resources Information Center
	National Institute of Education

U. S. Department of Health, Education,
and Welfare
Washington, D. C. 20202
Published monthly
Annual cost: $38.00
Available from 1966

Resources in Education provides the most recent information a-
bout documents available in the field of educational research.
The documents in RIE are prepared by a coordinating staff in
Washington, D. C. and 16 clearing houses located at universities
or with professional organizations across the country.   These
clearing houses are each responsible for a particular educational
area such as *teacher education; information resources; languages
and linguistics; and tests, measurement, and evaluation.*

The document résumés are arranged in numerical order by
ED number (ERIC accession number) and alphabetically by
clearing house prefix initials and acquisition number. Résumés
also provide information about price, availability, descriptors,
etc.

The subject index lists accession numbers and titles of documents under the major subjects that have been assigned to characterize their contents.   The subjects, which conform to those
presented in the Thesaurus of ERIC Descriptors, are in alphabetical order.

In performing subject searches of this abstract journal, researchers should refer to the Thesaurus of ERIC Descriptors.
Since *Motor Development* is a descriptor in the thesaurus, one
consults the subject index to find the accession number.   The
title is also provided here, so the user can judge the relevancy
of the document.   For example:

Motor Development
   Effects of Perceptual-Motor Training on Preschool
   Children: A Multivariate Approach
        ED 096 286

Also contained in RIE are author and institution indices. The first contains author, title, and accession number; the second, institution, title, and accession number. Finally, there is a list of descriptors which have been added to the thesaurus to define headings and cross-references.

Name:	**Social Sciences Citation Index (SSCI)**
Address:	Institute for Scientific Information
	325 Chestnut Street
	Philadelphia, Pa. 19106

Published triannually (cumulated annually)

Annual Cost: $1,250.00

Available from 1970

The *Social Sciences Citation Index* provides a complete indexing system to the literature of the social sciences. It indexes every article and significant editorial from every issue of over 1400 social sciences journals. SSCI also indexes 1200 selectively covered journals, from which it chooses only articles deemed relevant to social sciences.

Included in the SSCI are three separate but related indices: *The Citation Index, Permuterm Subject Index,* and *Source Index.*

Citation Index (SSCI)

This index shows which previously published items are being cited in current literature, who is doing the citing, and in which journals they are cited. This index can help the researcher to find out if certain works have been cited; if there are reviews on the subject; if the idea is original, etc.

Entries are arranged alphabetically by cited author. Following each item is a list of the current articles that have cited it, and these are also arranged alphabetically by authors. Special sections of the Citation Index cover articles that cite (1) anonymously authored items, and (2) those authored by an organization rather than an individual. *Cited* items can be books, articles, letters, theses, or any other type of material published at any time. *Citing* items are always articles published during the period being indexed.

Permuterm Subject Index (PSI)

The Permuterm Subject Index is a permuted title-word index to the journals processed for the *Social Sciences Citation Index*. In PSI every significant word in each title is paired with every other significant word in the same title. PSI is a natural language indexing system based on the language used by authors. To use PSI, one simply thinks of words and word pairs likely to appear in the titles of articles related to his or her topic of interest. An alphabetical check of these words then leads the searcher to the names of authors who have used the words in the titles of their articles. To obtain the full bibliographical reference, he can then look up the names of these authors in the Source Index.

A listing for motor development would appear as follows in the PSI:

```
MOTOR
Develop         -  Verbitsk, GI
Development  -  Adelson, E
             -  Ball, TS
             -  Bialer, I
             -  Chasey, WC
```

Source Index

The Source Index lists in alphabetical order every author of every source item processed for the SSCI. Beginning with the May-August 1974 issue, the list of references from each source item also appears in the Source Index. Under the author's name, source items for a particular year are listed in alphabetical order by journal title abbreviation. The information given includes co-authors, language code, title, volume, page, year, type of source item (e.g., editorial), and a number of references.

Used by itself, the Source Index is an excellent way to follow the work of specific authors and organizations. But it also supports the Citation and Permuterm Indices because the searcher must refer, by the author's names, back to the Source Index for a complete description of the articles located in either of the other indices.

Name:	**Index Medicus**
Address:	Chief Bibliographic Services Division
	National Library of Medicine
	8600 Rockville Pike
	Bethesda, Md. 20014

Published monthly
Annual Cost: $188.00
Available from 1960

Index Medicus coverage is limited to periodical literature. Symposia, congress proceedings, and similar materials are indexed only if they appear in periodicals. The content of each article is described by assigning terms selected from the National Library of Medicine's (NLM) Medical Subject Headings list (MeSH). This is a controlled vocabulary list of approximately 8500 technical terms used by the NLM. It should be examined by the user before he or she begins a search. In the cumulated *Index Medicus,* the MeSH is reprinted in its entirety.

Subject Section. Each article is assigned as many subject headings as are needed to describe the content adequately. The article appears in *Index Medicus* only under those subject headings which represent the most important concepts of the article. If the medical concept you have in mind is not a medical subject heading, you will need to find the MeSH equivalent. Thus, an article concerned with *motor development* is indexed under *motor*

skills with a cross-reference to the related term, *child development*. The user interested in one specific concept may find that
the broader term is also worth examining for articles of possible
interest. To find broader and narrower terms, refer to MeSH
Tree Structures. Each subject heading is grouped into one or
more of 14 subject categories including *diseases (C), organisms
(B),* and *psychiatry and psychology (F)*. *Motor skills* would be
found under *psychiatry and psychology* as *(F1) psychologic
mechanisms and processes*. A narrower term under *motor skills*
is *task performance and analysis*.

Author Section. References in the Author Section cite a maximum of three authors' names, and complete citations are printed
only under the first author's name. The second and third authors' names are cross-referenced to the first author.

Medical Reviews. The articles in this section represent surveys
of recent biomedical literature and include an abbreviation of
journal titles.

Name:	**Health, Physical Education, and Recreation**
	Microcard Bulletin
Address:	Microcard Publications
	School of Health, Physical Education, and Recreation,
	University of Oregon
	Eugene, Ore. 97403

Published irregularly

Annual cost:	No charge for Bulletin, but variable charges for the purchase of microcards

Available from 1949

The Microcard Publications project is conducted by the School of
Health, Physical Education, and Recreation at the University of
Oregon, as a nonprofit service to the professions involved. The
Bulletin emphasizes unpublished research materials (particularly

doctoral dissertations and masters' theses) and scholarly books now out of print. The microcard index for Volumes 1 and 2 (1949-1965, 1965-1972) is divided into subject matter topics and author indices. *Motor development* is a subject matter topic. For example, the following entry would be found under *motor development* in the subject matter index:

> Motor Development
> Effect of ball trajectory on catching skill,
> PE 807, Bruce

Located in the microcard title section would be the following information:

> PE 807 Bruce, Russell D. The effects of variations in ball trajectory upon catching performance of elementary school children, 1966, Doctor of Philosophy dissertation, University of Wisconsin. (143 pages, 4 cards, $1.80)

Microcard bulletins published since 1972 do not have a subject index, so from this point the user would have to make a page-by-page search for titles relating to motor development research.

Name:	**Completed Research in Health, Physical Education, and Recreation**
Address:	American Alliance for Health, Physical Education, and Recreation 1201 16th Street, N. W. Washington, D. C. 20036

Published annually
Annual Cost: $5.50
Available from 1959

Completed Research in Health, Physical Education, and Recreation is arranged in three parts: *I. Index, II. Bibliography*, and

III. Theses Abstracts. The index enables the reader to refer to items of completed research listed in Parts II and III, but is limited to subject headings and research topics. Indexing is not available by author.

Part II, the bibliography, lists published research, citing articles published in the 180 periodicals reviewed by the Committee for Completed Research. The listing is alphabetical with a number code and includes the author, title, volume, page (s), month, and year. Abstracts are not included.

Part III, Theses Abstracts, lists masters' and doctoral theses from institutions offering graduate programs in health, physical education, recreation, and allied areas. Most references are accompanied by abstracts of research, and all are number coded in alphabetical order according to the institution.

In performing subject searches here, researchers should use the subject index. Lists of coded numbers indicating research relating to motor development are simply located in the index under the heading, *motor development.*

Name:	**Abstracts of Research Papers**
Address:	American Alliance for Health,
	Physical Education and Recreation
	1201 16th Street
	Washington, D. C. 20036
Published annually	
Annual Cost:	$2.75

Abstracts of Research Papers includes abstracts, precisely submitted by the authors, of papers scheduled at the annual convention of the American Alliance for Health, Physical Education, and Recreation. An author index, but not a subject index, is included in each volume. Searching for motor development research requires a page-by-page title and abstract search, but usually the annual volume is less than 150 pages.

B

Creating a
Motor Development Laboratory

MARCELLA V. RIDENOUR

What are the options regarding the organization, facilities, resources, and activities of a motor development laboratory within
a university or college physical education program? The laboratory would be used by undergraduate and graduate students, and
educational professionals from the community. Its purpose
would be to facilitate both research and teaching related to the
motor development of young children. Above all, it would provide a center for the design, construction, and evaluation of unique and inexpensive equipment for use in motor development
programs and research projects.

In an effective motor development laboratory, emphasis
should be on *real* projects. Too frequently, students are required
only to draw or make models of motor development or play
equipment for young children—and drawings and models have
very limited application to the actual building and designing
of environments. In the real world there exists space, time, and
budget limitations as well as the skills required to build in medi-
ums involving masonry, carpentry and electronics. A motor development laboratory provides students with real situations both
for course projects and for independent study. These real situations may include tools, materials, and children, and will help
bridge the gap between a student's university training and his
later employment by a school, youth agency, or institution.

The structure and functions of the laboratory varies from
institution to institution. In one, the laboratory may emphasize experimental research, while another may emphasize teaching and applied research. A common element of all motor

development laboratories, however, is the provision of *space, tools, materials,* and *consultation* on the design of innovative motor development programs and research with infants and young children.

This appendix provides a brief description of the possible equipment and programs of a motor development laboratory. In fact, the last section describes possible projects which may be completed in the laboratory.

The time schedule of a motor development laboratory should be flexible enough to accomodate regularly scheduled classes (short and long-term), and consultation with laboratory specialists. Examples of activities requiring a reserved time period are:

1. *Undergraduate and graduate credit courses* with regularly scheduled laboratory time blocks. Courses in this category may be psychology of movement, motor development, perceptual motor development, or elementary physical education.

2. *Noncredit lecture series.* A regularly scheduled weekly seminar on proposed, ongoing, or completed research relating to motor development or motor learning may be scheduled as part of the regular laboratory activities.

3. *Symposia.* Approximately every 6 to 12 months a symposium may be scheduled drawing in both local specialists and national and international authorities in motor development. Announcement of the symposium could be sent to major universities and colleges and local preschool, elementary, and secondary agencies. A small fee charged participants would provide an honorarium and travel expenses for major speakers.

4. *Short courses.* Short courses could serve to present techniques, processes, or procedures to be used in motor development programs and experiments. Possible topics might be computer programming techniques applied to motor develop-

ment research, basic electronic instrumentation to record spatial and temporal characteristics of human movement, high-speed motion photographic techniques applied to motor development research, use of power tools to build climbing equipment for young children, and how to build ferroconcrete playground structures. The nature and scope of these and other short courses would be determined by the goals and priorities of the laboratory.

5. *Demonstration programs.* Frequently during the academic year, demonstration programs provide the opportunity for students to observe ongoing motor development programs. Examples of these would be a developmental motor education program for preschool children; motor stimulation programs for high-risk infants; or gymnastics instruction for 3-, 4-, and 5-year-old children.

Equipment and Materials

The key to a flexible laboratory is having an adequate workshop area where students and faculty can quickly assimilate materials— where they can build the needed equipment with minimal frustration and delay. Most motor development instruments can be designed and constructed for a fraction of the manufacturer's retail price. If the apparatus is for short-term use only, the components can easily be reassembled into future instruments. A basic workshop should include the following tools, supplies, materials, and library references:

1. *Hand tools.* Hammers, screwdrivers, squares, hand saws including a hack saw, plane, chisels, bench vise, C-clamps, manual miter box, folding steel saw horses, 50- and 100-feet wind-reel measuring tapes, wrench set, socket set, hex key set, rubber mallet, and files.

2. *Power tools.* Radial arm saw, portable circular saw, portable scroller sabre saw, reciprocating saw, power drills (3/8-inch reversible and cordless rechargeable ½-inch drills), belt sander with dust pick-up, shop vacuum, drill bits, and hole cutters.

3. *Electrical tools and instruments.* Portable rechargeable soldering pen, plug-in soldering gun, wire cutters, wire strippers, several time clocks accurate to .001 seconds, several prebuilt relay boxes, two pairs of prebuilt photoelectric cells, and long-armed microswitches.

4. *Outdoor playground building tools.* Large chain saw, assorted shovels, long-handled pick, concrete mixing boat, trowels and post hole diggers, water hoses and hoe.

5. *Supplies and materials.* Supplies and materials must be continuously replaced as used. Plywood sheets (4 x 6 feet, 3/8- and 5/8-inch thick), boards (2 x 4 inches, 1 x 6 inches, 10 feet long), dowel rods (4 feet long, 1 inch in diameter), nails, screws, nuts, bolts, electrical wiring, ropes, cords, twines, cement, gravel, sand, foam chips, foam pieces, pieces of clear plexiglass, masking tape, colored cloth tape, duct tape, polythene, steel wool, sandpaper, and long handled microswitches.

6. *Charge accounts and standing orders.* The laboratory workshop should be supplemented by the institution's physical plant or by private firms providing both services and supplies. Suggested supplementary agencies are carpentry, electronic, plumbing, and machine shops; and hardware, toy, and lumber stores.

7. *Workshop Library.* Listed below are examples of basic reference books that would strengthen a workshop library:

Ambercrombie, Stanley, *Ferrocement: Build with Cement, Sand, and Wire Mesh*, New York: Schocken Books, 1977.

Presents techniques for building structures with sand molds, covering with polythene and tape, three or four layers of wire mesh, followed by 3/4-inch-thick mixture of sand and cement. Techniques can easily be applied to playground building. Examples include a flower pot, garden sculpture, and dome.

Ashley, Clifford, *The Ashley Book of Knots,* Garden City, N. Y.: Doubleday, 1944.

Provides technical information for using knots. Reader must be able to apply technical information to practical playground projects.

Basic Hand Tools, U. S. Government Printing Office, Washington, D. C.: Division of Public Documents, 1963.

Describes the use of basic hand tools.

Campbell, R., *How to Work with Tools and Wood,* New York: Pocket Books, A Division of Simon and Schuster, 1952.

Presents a comprehensive introduction to wood tools, with 500 illustrations.

Design and Control of Concrete Mixes, Skokie, Ill.: Portland Cement Association.

Presents all aspects of quality control in mixing concrete.

Graumont, R. M., and Hensel, J., *Encyclopedia of Knots and Fancy Rope Work,* Cambridge, Md.: Cornel Maritime Press, 1952.

Provides diagrams and illustrations for all the knots you will need to construct rope ladders and cargo nets. Includes an extensive section on cargo nets. This book includes very complex macrame' that, when done on a large scale, could provide exciting movement experiences for young children.

Hogan, P., *Playgrounds for Free,* Boston: MIT Press, 1974.

Presents a series of photographs with a brief description of many free, recycled, or inexpensive playgrounds.

Inflatocookbook, Sausalito, Cal.:   Ant Farm (247 Gate 5 Road), 1972.

Describes the design and construction of inflatables which can be used for varied movement experiences for young children. These may resemble an immense water bed, slow motion trampoline, or squishy mountain.

Wagner, W. H., *Modern Carpentry,* South Holland, Ill.:   The Goodhead-Wilcox Co., Inc., 1976.

Presents carpentry in an easy-to-understand format.

Valkenburgh, V.   *Basic Electricity,* New York: Hayden Book Company, 1954, 5 volumes.

Presents basic electricity with graphic illustrations.

Valkenburgh, V.   *Basic Electronics,* New York: Hayden Book Company, 1959.

Presents basic electronics with graphic illustrations.

The word to summarize the ultimate workshop area is *flexibility,* supplemented by resources within the university and community.

If research is a basic goal of the motor development laboratory, tools are necessary for both movement analysis and subsequent data manipulation.   The tools for movement analysis are primarily photoinstruments.   Although other systems are available involving either electromyography or electrogonimetry, these systems frequently interfere with the natural movement pattern of a young child, because both require attaching recording instruments to the body with electrical cords to transfer data from the body to the receiving unit.   Other systems are being developed which may be superior to photoinstrumentation in that they will permit immediate input to and output from a computer system. These future systems will not involve cameras or films, but instead will use light and/or sound receivers. The future light systems involve electro-optical receivers which collect and analyze the light patterns from a series of small blinking LED lights attached to the body. They will also involve several audioreceivers to collect and analyze ultrasound originating from small transmitters attached to key body landmarks.

The purpose of a movement analysis is to record, store, and retrieve data describing a human body while it is motion. The usual procedure involves a two-dimensional analysis of human movement. The analyst takes either a photograph, a series of photographs, or a motion film of a moving event. Prior to photography, markers (½-inch black circles with a white dot in the center) are placed on major joints of the performer's body. Minimal clothes are worn so they do not hide the moving limbs or torso. If a film is used; after it has been developed, it is analyzed on a frame-by-frame projector. The analysis consists of measuring the horizontal and vertical location of the selected body markers. The measuring instruments are usually either a measuring stick and tracing paper, a set of calibrated moving vertical and horizontal crosshairs and a rear projection screen, or a pen with a special surface for film projection. Commercial instruments are available to project, analyze, and record data. Some of the instruments will provide key-punched or on-line computer input from the frame-by-frame film data.

Computer programs can be written to describe many movement characteristics of one performer or of a group of performers. Locomotor characteristics that have been described after limited computer programming (to manipulate the raw data) are: stride length, stride rate, ankle angle, knee angle, hip angle, and coordinated relationships between arms, feet, and head movements.

The basic equipment needed for photoinstrumentation of motion of infants and young children is:

1.   A 16mm motion camera with several
      lenses or telescopic lens, frame rate of
      64 frames per second, electric motor
      drive, and variable speed shutter. (The

frame rate of 64 frames per second will usually be too slow for motor learning and biomechanical studies with adults.)

2. A 35mm camera with optional motor drive for creating a series of photographs of one movement event. The camera should permit exposure times between several seconds and 1/1000 second.

3. A 16mm film projector with stop action and variable projection speed capabilities, and an appropriate screen.

4. A motion analyzer or digitizer.

5. 16mm cutting and splicing equipment.

6. A time clock for accurate description of the temporal characteristics of movement while filming young children.

The laboratory photography area may be supplemented by a university or commercial darkroom facility for developing film and enlarging negatives. A university or commercial key punch service usually can provide inexpensive and very accurate key punching of data and programs to be delivered to a central computer center.

Photoinstrumentation provides an excellent tool for recording and describing movement accurately, but without aid of a computer or semi-automatic film reader, it could be a very time-consuming process. The researcher should determine definite temporal or spatial characteristics to be recorded, and then select the photoinstrumentation procedure to meet his objectives.

Detailed information on photoinstrumentation procedures can be obtained from the following references:

Grieve, D. W., *et al.*, *Techniques for the Analysis of Human Movement,* Princeton, N. J.: Princeton Book Company, 1976.

Hay, J. G., *The Biomechanics of Sports Techniques,* Englewood Cliffs, N. J.: Prentice-Hall, 1973.

Miller, D. I., & Nelson, R. L., *Biomechanics of Sport,* Philadelphia: Lea and Febiger, 1973.

Plagenhoef, S., *Patterns of Human Motion—A Cinematographic Analysis*. Englewood Cliffs, N. J.: Prentice-Hall, 1971.

Proceedings of the International Biomechanical Conference, Baltimore, Md.: University Park Press, 1969, 1971, 1973, 1975

Frequent seminars on photoinstrumentation and movement are conducted by Visual Data Systems, 5617 West 63rd Place, Chicago, Ill. 60638. They usually include camera selection, lighting, qualitative film analysis, quantitative film analysis, 2- and 3-dimensional analysis, and references and publications relating to photoinstrumentation.

Physical Design

Usually the motor development laboratory will require about 1200 square feet, although a large closet adjacent to a gymnasium can be used. Figure B-1 represents a drawing of a larger room converted to a motor development laboratory. The ideal laboratory has a floor partially tiled, partially carpeted. The carpeted area is necessary for motor activities with prewalking infants, while the tile area can be used for performance of specific motor skills and for a more easily maintained workshop floor. The carpet should be dark so that the photographs and motion films of the infant can easily distinguish the infant with minimal clothes from his or her surroundings.

One of the laboratory walls could be painted flat black to serve as a background in filming studies of human movement. A series of horizontal and vertical white lines each 1 inch wide, may be painted on the wall at 3 foot intervals to assist with the quantitative and qualitative analysis of human movement. Near one of the corners on this wall could be a one-way window for observers.

The workshop area could be located on the opposite wall. The workshop may include a wall-length work counter with appropriate undercounter and overcounter cabinets. This wall and work area adjoins the noncarpeted section of the floor.

The third wall could have tables and benches which fold up when the entire floor space is needed for practice experiences and

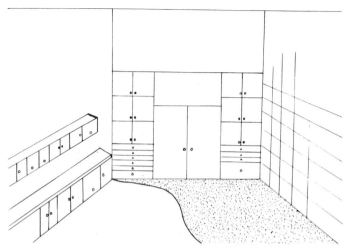

Figure B-1. Motor development laboratory.

research projects, and their seating or working capacity should be determined by class size.

Finally, the last wall may have ceiling-to-wall storage cabinets, 3 feet deep, on both sides of the double door entrance to the laboratory. A high ceiling with a grid of metal cross beams (for hanging experimental equipment apparatus) and temporal room dividers (cloth or wooden) may be desirable too. Also, a 15-foot overhead track with moving overhead camera mount may be incorporated into the ceiling.

Although a large physical environment is best for the motor development laboratory, a laboratory may be successfully operated from a combination of offices, basements, closets, and hallways. At most institutions cooperative arrangements can be made with other departments to "borrow" equipment and laboratory space.

Selected Motor Development Design Projects

The six motor development design projects selected here exemplify potential laboratory projects. Each description includes a summary of the laboratory's involvement as well as the purpose and structure of the specific project.

Climbing Boxes and Sliding Board

The boxes and sliding board (see Figure B-2) could be built for an indoor movement education program involving children between 1 and 5 years old. The purpose of the sliding board and boxes is to provide climbing, crawling, and sliding experiences normally not available in the child's home environment. The boxes and sliding board can be constructed from boards (2 x 4 inches), plywood, and sheet metal roofing (for the slide) by using the portable circular and sabre saw, a hammer, and a square. The construction procedure involves building frame boxes from the boards, then nailing on the plywood sheets with precut holes. The sides of the boxes can be painted with bright primary colors.

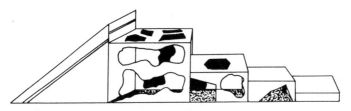

Figure B-2. Climbing boxes and sliding board.

Wooden Spool Mill House

A spool mill house can be built for an outdoor motor development area of a day care center. The purpose of the spool house (see Figure B-3) is to provide vertical climbing experiences to preschool children. Local wire companies will usually donate the spools free. Although this design involves stacked spools, it can easily be changed according to the movement desired, outcome, age of children, and number and size of available spools.

Wooden cross pieces may be placed in the spools to encourage climbing. Some of the larger spools have two levels inside; in this case, large circular holes can be cut with a reciprocating saw to permit the children to move freely between the four inside levels. Windows and doors may be made in the spool sides with the reciprocating saw. Holes 1¼ inches wide may be drilled with the power saw around the edges of the walk on the upper story. Free, used 1-inch pipe is then dropped into the holes to prevent children from falling from the exterior ledge. The exterior of the spools should be painted with exterior primer followed by two coats of exterior house paint. The inside can be painted with exterior primer and interior/exterior primary colors.

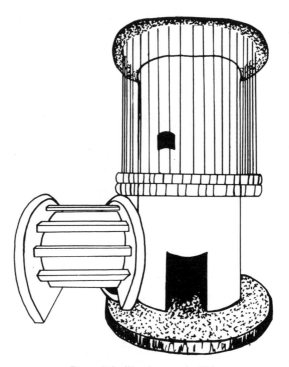

Figure B-3. Wooden spool mill house.

Telephone Pole Sliding Board

A telephone pole sliding board for an outdoor motor development area of a day care center can also be constructed easily. Here the purpose is to provide the preschool children with climbing and sliding experiences. Start by obtaining damaged telephone poles from a salvage lot of an electric utility company. The stainless steel sheet metal may be purchased from a sheet metal distributor. Place the "climbing poles" 18 inches into the ground and then secure them together with 100 feet of metal strapping and nails. The telephone pole frame for the slide can then be attached to the vertical poles with long nuts and bolts so that it looks like Figure B-4.

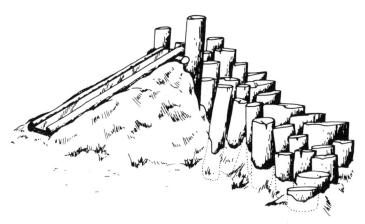

Figure B-4. Telephone pole sliding board.

Crazy Stairs

"Crazy stairs" may be used in an indoor movement education program involving children between 1 and 5 years old, and they can provide the children with several creeping, stepping, and climbing experiences. The center box for the stairs (see Figure B-5) is constructed from plywood. The steps are made to have heights and widths varying on each side of the box. The front stairs have variable slopes and a ladder is used on the fourth side of the box. All steps have plywood boards under the stairs to prevent the child from falling after an inaccurate step. The tools and materials required to complete the project are boards, plywood, angle brackets, hammer and nails, screwdriver and screws, and primary interior paint.

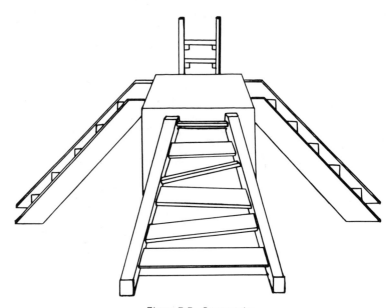

Figure B-5. Crazy stairs.

Jumping Accuracy Box

The purpose of the jumping accuracy box is to permit the experimenter quantitatively to examine the accuracy of first-grade children as they attempt to jump on a series of foot steps. Plexiglass tables combine with mirrors to permit a 16mm camera to record jumping accuracy of the child from *underneath* the table. Later film analysis is done by tracing the outline of the target foot and outline of the child's foot. Jumping accuracy is recorded as a percentage of the area of the child's foot on the target foot. Of course, target footprints must be adjusted to the foot size of each child. The only drawback in this two-camera technique is that it records data on the *outcome of* the movement rather than the *process.* An additional 16mm camera recording the child's arm, leg, head, and torso movements, however, can provide continuous recordings of the movement process. By doing so, it permits the examination of both the movement process and movement accuracy. Figure B-6 diagrams the jumping accuracy box.

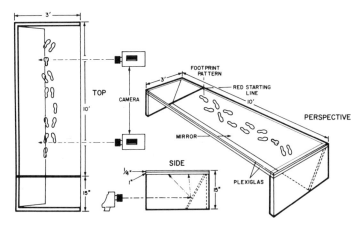

Figure B-6. Jumping accuracy box.

Locomotor Accuracy Box and Walking Under a Stick

The purpose of the locomotor accuracy box is to permit the experimenter to examine quantitatively the accuracy of the first-grade children locomoting through a box with several spatial restrictions both over and under the subject. The box may have between one and thirty horizontal poles to restrict the child's locomotion. The child is instructed to move through the box without touching the poles. When the child touches a spring-suspended pole, a low voltage relay box activates a continuous error timer.

A total error score, representing movement outcome, is recorded when the locomotion through the box is completed. Figure B-7 diagrams the locomotor accuracy project. Adding a 16mm camera to record the body movements of the child can provide additional, continuous information on the movement process of the first-grade children.

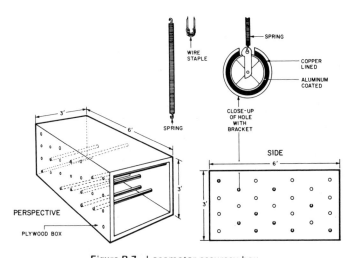

Figure B-7. Locomotor accuracy box.

A less complex motor skill, walking under one stick, also provides more information describing the child's movement performance if a 16mm film record of the task is used to create the movement description. This technique provides information on both movement process and movement outcome. Figure B-8 illustrates a child moving under one stick.

Through projects such as these, a motor development laboratory can meet the needs of children, students, researchers, and teaching faculty associated with the laboratory. Laboratory components such as those suggested here can adapt to many situations. Certainly, the six selected projects should not be interpreted as projects that should be built by all laboratories. There are merely illustrations of the *potential for flexibility* in the laboratory described. Only the needs of the faculty and students in your particular institution will determine your own laboratory projects.

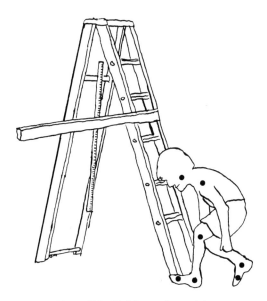

Figure B-8. Walking under a stick.

Indexes

Subject Index

Author Index